The Fat-Burning Bible

The Fat-Burning Bible

28 Days of Foods, Supplements, and Workouts That Help You Lose Weight

Mackie Shilstone

WILEY

John Wiley & Sons, Inc.

Published by John Wiley & Sons, Inc., Hoboken, New Jersey
Published simultaneously in Canada

The author gratefully acknowledges the permission granted by the following to include their work: "Signs and Symptoms of Hypothyroidism" questionnaire (chap. 6) by Dr. Charles Mary III; "Quality-of-Life Assessment of Human Growth Hormone Deficiency" questionnaire (chap. 6) by Mario R. McNally, MD; the stress questionnaires and solutions for stress (chap. 7) are used by permission of the National Mental Health Association, Alexandria, Va.; "PAR-Q and You" questionnaire (chap. 13) is reprinted from the 2004 revised version of the Physical Activity Readiness Questionnaire. "PAR-Q and You" is a copyrighted, pre-exercise screen owned by the Canadian Society for Exercise Physiology; illustrations (chap. 4) by Barbara Seide; photographs (chap. 13) by Toby Armstrong.

For general information about our other products and services, please contact our Customer Care Department within the United States at (800) 762-2974, outside the United States at (317) 572-3993 or fax (317) 572-4002.

Wiley also publishes its books in a variety of electronic formats. Some content that appears in print may not be available in electronic books. For more information about Wiley products, visit our web site at www.wiley.com.

Library of Congress Cataloging-in-Publication Data:
Shilstone, Mackie.
    The fat-burning bible : 28 days of foods, supplements, and workouts that help you lose weight / Mackie Shilstone.
        p.   cm.
    Includes bibliographical references and index.
    ISBN 0-471-65529-5 (cloth)
    1. Weight loss. 2. Adipose tissues. 3. Metabolism. I. Title.
    RM222.2.S52678   2004
    613.7—dc22   2004014377

Printed in the United States of America

10   9   8   7   6   5   4   3   2

Contents

Foreword

by Kathy Smith

I'm convinced that being overfat is one of the most serious problems our society faces. I've worked with countless women over the years and I've seen how it can destroy a person's health, undermine one's self-esteem, and drastically limit one's enjoyment and participation in all that life has to offer. And yet even after three decades in the fitness industry, it still surprises me how much confusion there is surrounding the best way to eat and exercise. This confusion is only made worse by the dizzying array of shortcuts and quick fixes out there and by the fact that most people just don't have the time or energy to sort out truth from fiction.

Here then to the rescue is Mackie Shilstone's *The Fat-Burning Bible*— one of the most comprehensive nutritional and exercise programs I've ever encountered. This groundbreaking work is sure to be a powerful tool in the hands of anyone wanting to lose excess body fat while increasing his or her knowledge about this complex subject.

As the Ochsner Clinic Foundation's Performance Enhancement Expert, Mackie is well versed in the science of nutrition, fitness, and sports medicine. What's more, Mackie's metabolic prescriptions offered in this book are based upon his nearly thirty years of experience working with over three thousand top athletes and many thousands of ordinary women and men.

Mackie isn't kidding when he calls his book a "bible"—indeed, its scope and degree of detail are remarkable. While we've all heard the standard one-liners on key topics like insulin resistance and cholesterol, Mackie's book explores the underlying science to give you the deeper story. From how to interpret your lipid profile to disease markers, HGH, whey proteins, and a long list of others—many of the topics covered are things I've learned about and discussed with my *own* doctors. Still, I've never seen them explained more clearly and accessibly than in this book. Through careful organization of the material, Mackie's explanations have the miraculous power to simultaneously provide more detail *and* a simplified understanding.

If you're like me, knowing the why behind the what is a key factor in staying motivated and developing consistency with a program. Consistency in turn is the key to success. *The Fat-Burning Bible* will take you as far as you want to go toward a thorough understanding of human physiology as it relates to weight loss—and it will show you how to use that knowledge to get results.

I've spent my professional life sounding the call for lifestyle change. That's why it's such a pleasure to have another authoritative voice joining that call, especially one backed by such extensive research and armed with such practical solutions.

Obesity is becoming the number one disease in North America. The powerful exercise, nutritional, and stress-reducing strategies in this book are one sure step toward a cure.

Preface

I have always tried to be an innovator instead of simply copying others. In my health and fitness work I've striven to be on the cutting edge as opposed to the cutting room floor. One of the things I learned when I got my MBA in business is that if you want to succeed you've got to have a model. That's what I've done in this book and in my two others, *Lose Your Love Handles* and *Maximum Energy for Life,* as I've given readers a clear, easy-to-follow model of a good health and lifestyle program. In this book I provide understandable, tried-and-true strategies to either remain slim or to lose dangerous body fat. In this way, I am empowering you to avoid many of the diseases that are decimating the lives of literally millions of Americans.

Over the years, my work has been about stepping out boldly and using recognized, leading-edge health technologies to create success in my clients, whether they are world-class athletes or ordinary men and women from all walks of life. In 1985, I made history by helping Michael Spinks to be the first light heavyweight to become a heavyweight champion when he took the title from Larry Holmes. In March 2003, I used similar techniques to help Roy Jones Jr., the light heavyweight champion, to successfully defeat John Ruiz, the World Boxing Association heavyweight champion. Once again, we did the impossible. And, I might add, in twenty years no one else has duplicated these efforts.

The exercise and nutritional models presented in this book work. They have enabled athletes to extend their careers far beyond the norm. They have allowed men and women suffering from morbid obesity and life-threatening diseases to extend their lives. This program has given thousands of people a quality of life, health, and performance far beyond their wildest expectations.

The Next Wave of Disease Management

For years you have been reading about the three most prevalent diseases in the United States: heart disease, type 2 diabetes, and cancer. And for twenty-seven years I have been writing about and treating these deadly illnesses. While planning this book I asked myself, What common link do all of these diseases have? The answer is easy: they are most likely to develop when we put on excess fat with age.

In *Maximum Energy for Life,* cardiologist Chip Lavie made the startling statement that 95 percent of all heart disease is preventable. We gave you the facts and the program to prove it. In this book I am taking this concept one step further. I believe that obesity should be named the number one preventable disease in this country, because almost all major health problems have overweight or obesity at their core. Obesity is responsible for a whole constellation of problems generally known as heart disease: high cholesterol, hypertension, heart attack, and stroke. It is the number one cause of adult-onset type 2 diabetes. A recent landmark study involving 90,000 cancer-free individuals designed to examine the relationship between cancer and fat found that the risk for *all* types of cancer was increased by being overfat or obese.

It is far easier to avoid disease than to control it. If you contract diabetes, you're always going to have it. You can only learn strategies to manage it. If you allow your cardiovascular health to degenerate to the point where you suffer a heart attack, you'll always have the potential for another heart attack; you will just have to develop a lifestyle plan to minimize a recurrence.

What This Book Can Do for You

This book not only gives you tools to help you to evaluate how overfat you are and what diseases you are at risk for, it gives you a strategic plan to take off the excess fat and keep it off. Here is some of the important fat-loss information you will receive from this book.

1. Changing a relationship with food is not like changing a relationship to drug addiction. I can't tell a person who is morbidly obese, "You'll never be able to eat again for the rest of your life." That's impossible. But in this book I can teach you to transform food from an enemy into an ally by explaining how it works in the body. The food program in *The Fat-Burning Bible* is not only delicious but will never leave you hungry.

2. People often ask me, "Is all fat bad?" No, it is not. Everyone has to have a certain amount of body fat to survive. But there are healthy

and unhealthy body fat percentages. Most important, there are healthy and unhealthy ways for fat to be distributed in the body. A normal man carries his fat above the waist. A normal woman carries hers in the hips and buttocks area. When your fat crosses the line and your body begins to take on the fat pattern of the opposite gender, then you have developed a potentially dangerous configuration known as a reverse fat pattern. This book shows you how to identify that pattern and how to eat in a way that will help burn fat and normalize where you carry your fat weight.

3. Studies have shown that women burn more fat at low to moderate levels of exercise intensity and men at moderate to high levels of exercise intensity. The exercise program in this book is designed to capitalize on these findings to help you boost your metabolism and achieve maximum fat loss for the time invested. During the basic four-week Fat-Burning Metabolic Fitness Exercise Plan, you will be performing 300 minutes of specially designed exercise per week, six days a week. If you wish to capitalize on your newfound metabolic efficiency and fat-burning capacity and lose even more weight, I offer you two more four-week programs that decrease in time but increase in intensity. In the second month, you will only need to exercise for 260 minutes per week, five days per week, and by the third month you will only need 200 minutes four days a week. My maintenance program, which is 150 minutes a week of moderate exercise, will keep you slim for life.

4. If you faithfully follow the Metabolic Fitness Plan, in as little as four weeks you will see a dramatic improvement in your overall appearance. You will lose an average of 14 to 16 pounds of scale weight in one month. For each pound lost, you should lose an average of three-quarters of an inch in your total body measurements. You will drop 0.75 percent of body fat/week. (If you continue into the third month, you will lose 1.5 percent body fat/week.) If you are a woman, you will drop two to three dress sizes in one month. If you are a man, you will see 2 to 4 inches disappear from your waistline.

5. If you choose to go to your doctor and get a lipid profile, you will most likely see an improvement in your total cholesterol, HDL (good cholesterol), triglycerides, and glucose. While heredity plays a part in the lipid profile—for example, high cholesterol runs in some families—studies have shown that people can control approximately 70 percent of hereditary factors through lifestyle.

6. If you suffer from imbalances in your levels of human growth hormone, thyroid, testosterone, and estrogen, you will see dramatic improvement in your hormonal profile in as little as four weeks.

7. Fifty percent of our children are obese or overweight and a significant number of kids are already experiencing major health problems such as high blood pressure, type 2 diabetes, deformities of the hips and knees, asthma, premature puberty, increased triglycerides, high cholesterol, and decreased levels of HDL. When an airplane is in trouble, parents are told to put on their oxygen mask so that they can help their children. The only way that we are going to save our kids is to put on the mask—to take responsibility for developing healthy nutritional and exercise patterns ourselves.

This book will give you powerful strategies to deal with fat accumulation as you age. As fat-related health problems spiral out of control in our society, the knowledge I am offering you here can literally save your life. If you are just beginning to put on fat, it can reverse this dangerous trend and keep you from succumbing to diseases prematurely in your thirties and forties.

What Is Unique about This Book

This book offers some unique benefits. There is a serious health care literacy gap in this country. While some of the cutting-edge information offered here exists in published form, the majority of it is written in dry, complicated language in scientific journals. As a member of Governor-elect Kathleen Blanco's transition team for the Department of Health and Hospitals and the Board of Directors of the National Mental Health Association, one of the things that I have learned is that you must take health care to the people in a form that they can easily digest. My collaborator, Joy Parker, and I have worked long and hard to take difficult scientific concepts and distill them into language that readers can understand, relate to, and effectively apply in their daily lives. We have tried to make this book as clear, helpful, and motivational as possible.

This is the first book ever written for the general public that effectively addresses the concept of the reverse fat pattern: the deadly effect of body fat that accumulates in an area of the body where it presents the greatest danger of disease. Being overfat or having excess fat in the wrong places has a great deal to do with imbalances in the sex hormones, testosterone and estrogen, as well as in human growth hormone, thyroid function, and the many kinds of hormones that affect fat storage and utilization. This book is one of the first to offer questionnaires to help you realize when your own hormones are working against you. It also discusses how the hormonal changes that occur with menopause and andropause can cause you to become overfat and tells you how exercise and nutrition can help rebalance these hormones.

This is the first book to recognize that men and women get the most benefit from exercise by doing their workouts at different intensities. As you will see, this is also related to how men's and women's bodies utilize hormones differently to effectively process food as energy or to store it as fat.

How This Book Is Set Up

Part one of this book is meant to educate you about several key concepts:

- The health risks of being overfat
- The role that metabolism plays in fat gain and loss
- The dangers of the reverse fat pattern and the hormonal differences in men and women
- The changes that occur with menopause and andropause and how to ease into this transition so that you can pass through it as easily as possible

Beginning with part two, this book replicates the way I run my Fat-Burning Metabolic Fitness Plan at the Mackie Shilstone Center for Performance Enhancement and Lifestyle Management at the Ochsner Clinic Foundation in New Orleans. It provides several self-assessment questionnaires that will help you to evaluate common health markers such as Body Mass Index, waist measurement, waist-to-hip ratio, percentage of body fat, total cholesterol, LDL (bad cholesterol), HDL (good cholesterol), triglycerides, glucose, human growth hormone levels, and thyroid function. I have also added a chapter on stress, which includes stress evaluation questionnaires and guidelines developed by the National Mental Health Association. Part two describes my Fat-Burning Metabolic Fitness Nutritional Plan, which includes delicious low-glycemic meal plans and recipes developed by my nutritionist, Molly Kimball, and chef, Mark Gilberti.

Part three outlines the benefits of exercise and the Fat-Burning Metabolic Fitness Exercise Plan. This program is made up of four distinct types of exercise. In the basic four-week program on days 1, 3, and 5 you will be doing 10 minutes of circuit/resistance exercises to increase metabolism and 50 minutes of steady-state cardio to increase your fat-burning capacity. On days 2, 4, and 6 you will be doing 10 minutes of core exercises to increase your metabolic rate and maximize fat loss in the central/abdominal area. You will follow these core exercises with 30 minutes of interval training to increase metabolic capacity. This totals 300 minutes per week of exercise. Part four provides you with a daily four-week self-evaluation guide to help you track your progress.

If you wish to capitalize on the increased metabolism and fat-burning ability of this four-week program, you may follow up with two additional four-week modules with a decreased amount of time investment and an increased level of intensity. I also provide you with a 150-minute/week moderate-intensity maintenance program that will keep you fit and slim for life.

This book represents the legacy of my twenty-seven years of helping clients to lose fat and improve their health. It presents state-of-the-art research in an accessible form, giving you all the tools you need to begin taking charge of your health. It gives me great pleasure to share this information with you. I wish you all the best as you read and utilize this material. I know that if you faithfully follow this program, you will have the same great level of success as thousands of others before you.

Acknowledgments

I would like to thank the following people for their invaluable help with this book:

My loving wife, Sandy, and my sons, Scott and Spencer, for their patience and understanding in helping me to fulfill this dream, my fourth book.

My friend and collaborator, Joy Parker, who over the years has continued to support my work, give me her personal insights, and translate my ideas and thoughts into easy-to-understand, applicable information that people have embraced for years to make their lives better. Without her words, this book would simply be an unfulfilled dream.

My literary agent, Bonnie Solow, for successfully helping me to bring this book into realization and for continuing to believe in me and what I do.

Tom Miller, my editor, for investing in my work for a second time and for having the vision to publish books that fulfill vital and specific areas of health care needs. I believe our books will go down in posterity as guides for effectively handling the major diseases in our health care system today.

Kellam Ayers, his executive assistant, for taking my numerous phone calls with a pleasant attitude and finding the answers.

Devra K. Nelson, our superb senior production editor, for her keen eye, patience, and helpfulness.

Yvonne Rocca and Tracy Moore, the models who posed for the exercise pictures.

My executive assistant, Kim Cummins, for her patience, friendship, and help in maintaining the manuscript throughout all of its many incarnations.

My nutritionist, Molly Kimball, for the fabulous work she did on the nutrition section of this book.

Mark Gilberti, food and beverage director of the Elmwood Fitness Center, for his help on the Mackie Meal recipes.

Ken Kachtik, general manager of the Elwood Fitness Center, for his continued support of my program.

Cardiologist Chip Lavie, MD, and Richard Milani, MD, codirectors of the Heart and Vascular Institute at the Ochsner Clinic Foundation, for their guidance and for naming me director of health and fitness at the institute.

Cameron Emerson, MD, obstetrician and gynecologist, for her feedback on menopause.

The National Mental Health Association for allowing us to use their stress and depression questionnaires and solutions, and for giving me a position on their board of directors.

Endocrinologist Mario McNally, MD, of the Touro Infirmary Hospital, for his help on human growth hormone and testosterone.

Chuck Mary III, MD, and James Carter, MD, DrPH, for their invaluable information on thyroid and human growth hormone.

Kathleen Wilson, MD, for her help with certain fine points of medicine.

Gerry Provance, DC, my chiropractor, for assisting me with the floor-based core exercises.

The doctors, nurses, and staff of the Ochsner Clinic Foundation for their continuing support.

Rachel Welp and Brian Picou for maintaining the statistics on my clients in the comprehensive weight-loss program at Elmwood Fitness Center.

Douglas Daniels, Bo Walker, Melinda Mabile, and Kim Cummins for adhering to the program and allowing me to use their success stories in this book.

Barbara Seide, my illustrator, who created the body measurement drawings for this book.

Physical therapist Genevieve Borne for her input in designing the home dumbbell exercise program.

The people at the Discovery Health Channel for their belief in my work.

Beth Salmon, executive editor, and the staff of *Let's Live* magazine for their continuing support and showcasing of my program.

The New Orleans Police Department for giving me the ability to fine-tune my program while benefiting their officers.

All the participants in my comprehensive weight-loss program at the Elmwood Fitness Center.

Sincere thanks to my friend Barry Goldman, MD, medical director of our Comprehensive Weight Management Program at the Ochsner Clinic Foundation, for making our program safe and medically sound.

What You Need to Know about Your Own Fat Pattern and Metabolic Fitness

1

Learn the Health Risks Associated with Excess Body Fat

Learn the Difference between Male and Female Fat Patterns

Where you carry your weight has serious health ramifications. The most dangerous type of weight is core body fat (abdominal obesity). People who carry weight more evenly distributed over their entire bodies are less at risk for disease than those who follow the more classic fat distribution patterns. Unfortunately, most men and women store excess weight above and below the waistline where it hurts the body the most.

For a variety of reasons, including hormones and metabolic processes that affect fat storage in particular areas of the body, when men and women first begin to gain weight, they do not store it in the same place. A typical overweight man looks like an apple. He carries his weight above the waist, resulting in the classic bulging abdomen, also known as the beer belly. A typical overweight woman carries her fat below the waist in the hips and the buttocks, resulting in a pear-shaped silhouette.

When obesity sets in, people often develop a reverse fat pattern. A man will not only have a huge belly but will start putting on considerable weight below the waist in the hips and buttocks. Women will not only store fat below the waist but will carry a large amount of abdominal fat, turning them into an apple shape. While being overweight increases health risks, crossing over into a reverse fat pattern is a move toward serious health risks.

Where Do You Carry Your Weight?

Where do you carry your weight? Before you read any further, do a quick visual evaluation of your fat pattern. Put on a swimsuit, stand in front of a full-length mirror, and take a look at where your body stores fat. Be honest about what you see. Does your weight distribution follow the classic male or female pattern? Or have you already crossed over into a high-risk reverse fat pattern? Have someone take pictures of you from the front, back, and side. Put them up someplace where you can see them every day such as on your bathroom mirror or refrigerator door. These pictures will become your motivation to stick with this program, and you will use them to evaluate your amazing progress as you drop inches and lose body fat.

When I first started my Fat-Burning Metabolic Fitness Plan, I would have someone videotape a "before" of my clients as they made a 360-degree turn. Then, four, eight, and twelve weeks later we would make a video record of the "afters" and compare the results. You may wish to create some sort of visual record as well, since it really shows you how dramatically your body can change in a relatively short amount of time. Kim Cummins, my executive assistant whose incredible makeover appeared in a recent article of *Let's Live* magazine, literally cried when she saw herself on film because she hadn't realized how much weight she had really gained. "I never realized how fat my face had become. It really shocked me."

Melinda Mabile, another participant in the *Let's Live* makeover, was delighted to see the difference in her before and after pictures. Even though Melinda did not lose a great deal of scale weight, she lost a significant amount of inches over her entire body and 7.8 percent body fat. Her waistline slimmed down noticeably. Her posture improved dramatically from month to month, along with her overall energy level. I watched her develop a vibrancy and sparkle—an attractiveness that comes from greater health and metabolic vitality. Melinda told me that she has never felt better in her life.

The Answer: Metabolic Fitness

If you find that you are overfat and suffering from a sluggish metabolism or that you have developed a reverse fat pattern, don't despair. Over the years I have helped thousands of men and women to lose fat, get in shape, balance their hormones, improve their blood chemistry, and increase their energy level. The four-week program in this book is guaranteed to help you not only lose unwanted fat but to dramatically improve your internal body chemistry—your cholesterol, triglycerides, blood sugar, hormonal balance, and thyroid function. And it will prolong the quality and length of your life. I also offer two additional four-week Fat-Burning Metabolic Fitness Exercise Modules and a Maintenance Plan. After four weeks on the basic program, I have found that most people have lost so much fat and increased their metabolism so dramatically that they wish to cash in on their newfound gains and go even further.

In over twenty-five years of work with thousands of top athletes, as well as nonathletic men and women, I have discovered that increasing metabolic fitness is the secret to losing body fat and lowering disease risk factors. My Fat-Burning Metabolic Fitness Plan is based on three tiers:

1. Fat-Burning Metabolic Fitness Self-Evaluation: an evaluation to learn how to honestly assess where you are on the fitness scale by measuring factors such as Body Mass Index, body measurements (including the all-important waist measurement), percent of body fat, and blood work, hormonal balance, and stress levels
2. Fat-Burning Metabolic Fitness Nutritional Plan: a low-glycemic meal plan to increase metabolism, reduce body fat, and boost energy levels
3. Fat-Burning Metabolic Fitness Exercise Plan: a gender-specific (intensity management) exercise system designed to trim inches of unwanted fat

Many fat-loss books give nutritional guidelines but do not feature the kind of high-powered exercise program that I offer in this book. But studies clearly show that eating right must be coupled with exercising right to really pay off. A recent study done by the Human Nutrition Program and published in the *Journal of Nutritional Biochemistry* clearly proves that while dieting is more effective in causing weight loss, exercise is more effective in reducing fat and building metabolically active lean body mass.

Remember, the choices you make in the area of lifestyle, nutrition, and exercise count toward 75 percent of your health profile. *And it is never too late to start improving your health.* If you are willing to follow the Fat-Burning Metabolic Fitness Plan set forth in this book, I can guarantee that you will soon be feeling and looking better than you ever have in your life.

2

The Six Facts You Must Know about Metabolism

To understand how my Fat-Burning Metabolic Fitness Plan works, you must first understand what is meant by the word *metabolism*. Metabolism is the sum total of all the chemical and physiological changes that take place within the body. This includes the transformation of food into energy, the growth and repair of muscle and bone tissue, and the creation of enzymes and hormones. The basal metabolic rate (BMR) accounts for about 70 percent of daily energy expenditure. The amount of energy required to digest and utilize food makes up 5 to 10 percent of daily energy output, and the energy expended in physical activity uses an additional 20 to 30 percent.

North Americans spend a total of $30 billion on commercial weight-loss programs and $6 billion on weight-loss products per year. At any given time, 25 percent of all men and 40 percent of all women are on some kind of diet. Yet we are still an overweight and obese society because we have many misconceptions about the metabolic processes that cause people to gain and lose body fat.

While it's true that almost any weight-loss regimen will cause you to lose pounds in the short run, the real issue is if you will be able to keep them off in the long run. Unfortunately, most diets fail the test of time. According to the American College of Sports Medicine, people gain back 67 percent of their lost weight within one year and the rest within five years.

Understanding Your Metabolism

To really understand how your metabolism works and how to make it work for you, there are six important facts you must keep in mind.

Fact #1: Fat Storage Is a Natural Survival Mechanism

The body's ability to efficiently store fat began as a survival mechanism when our human ancestors were hunter-gatherers. Up until the development of agriculture ten thousand years ago, human beings lived in an environment that had no quick and easy sources of food. Early humans needed some kind of physical means to store energy so that they could do the exhausting work of hunting down large animals, sometimes over great distances, running down smaller swift animals, and walking many miles daily to gather nuts, vegetables, grains, and fruits. This energy took the form of extra body fat.

While each person has a different ideal percentage of body fat depending on gender and frame size, generally an average healthy body fat is 18–22 percent for women and 15–17 percent for men.

Fact #2: Eating Too Little Can Slow Down Your Metabolism

Eating too few calories for the efficient functioning of your metabolism ultimately results in more stored fat. This might sound like a contradiction, but eating a calorically deprived diet over a long period of time actually causes the body to begin to hang on to the fat supplies it has and even add to them. Because a steady supply of food was not guaranteed to our hunter-gatherer forebears, the body developed the added ability to slow down the metabolism and store extra fat during periods of famine. If we did not have this ability, we would not have survived the lean times.

This is the primary reason that very low-calorie or starvation diets do not work in the long run. Almost everyone who has ever been on a calorically deprived diet knows that at first the pounds just melt off. But eventually you reach a plateau where you stop losing weight, no matter how hard you try. That is your body's natural fat-storing survival mechanism kicking in.

Recent studies have even shown an unexpected link between chronic caloric deprivation and obesity. Research conducted by Cornell University and the University of California at Davis have shown the connections between obesity, hunger, and poverty: poor women who periodically go without food so that their children can eat are often obese. The more often you starve yourself to try and lose weight, the slower and less efficient your metabolism will become.

In 1993 I had a client who was a former heavyweight boxing champion who would always be 25 to 45 pounds overweight going into our training camps. Each time we prepared him for a fight, he would be losing the same weight over and over again. This meant that we would have to prolong the usual six-week training period to about three months, which often brought us close to the edge of training burnout. It was a tremendous waste of time and resources to train a quarter of a year because of a simple weight issue.

On one occasion we had been training hard for two weeks and my client had not lost a single pound. This was a serious problem because the fight was only six weeks away. Thinking that low thyroid function might be the cause of his inability to lose weight, my doctor ordered a thyroid test, but the test came back normal.

At this time in my career, I had begun reading studies on metabolism. I consulted with the doctor we were using for this program, and he and I decided to run a simple metabolic activity test on our client. The test results showed that his metabolic rate had been slowed by 30 percent. We discovered the reason was that he wasn't following the food plan we had given him to help him lose weight and support the intense physical activity of his training program. Thinking it would help him to lose weight faster, he wasn't eating breakfast and was skimping on lunch. The opposite had occurred. He was tired in training and his body was hanging on to its fat supplies because it thought there was a famine going on. In other words it was slowing down his metabolic rate. At first it was difficult for us to convince him that he had to eat more to lose weight because it went against what he perceived as logic. But as soon as he began eating the proper number of calories and nutrients, he saw the pounds begin to come off.

In his book *Turn Up the Heat: Unlock the Fat-Burning Power of Your Metabolism,* nutritionist and champion bodybuilder Philip Goglia points out that we are a consistently underfed society: "I have found that most of the people who come to me with weight and health problems are usually *already* ingesting *far fewer calories* than they should in order to efficiently fuel their bodies. Therefore, their metabolism, the body's calorie-burning furnace, is already running 25 percent to 60 percent below its ideal metabolic-efficiency level. In turn, the body is storing much of the limited amounts of food these individuals eat as fat and wasting muscle tissue as an adaptive mechanism to create an alternative energy source."

You have to eat a certain amount of calories per day to lose body fat and preserve and build lean muscle mass. Eating too few calories can even cause your body to cannibalize its own lean muscle to get the nutrients needed for survival.

Fact #3: What You Eat Is as Important as How Much You Eat

Longevity studies have shown the importance of not only eating the right number of calories to support your metabolism but eating low-glycemic nutrient-dense calories to prolong the length, health, and quality of your life. For some this might indeed mean having to cut back on calories. But for most this won't be the case.

Our ancestors evolved by eating a diet of complex carbohydrates (high-fiber grains that took a long time to digest), lean protein, and fresh fruits and vegetables. In our current culture of processed foods, low-nutrition junk foods, and supersized meals, a person can go for weeks without eating a single piece of fresh produce. Because of large-scale, single-crop agribusiness, which picks most produce before it has even ripened so that it can be shipped to supermarkets hundreds or even thousands of miles away, we end up eating almost no fresh, ripe fruits and vegetables. In addition, our food is grown in soil so depleted in minerals that we get little nutritional value from it.

It does not help that we live in a culture that fears fats and carbohydrates. Most of the popular diet plans restrict one of these food groups.

Fear of Carbohydrates
People avoid carbohydrates because they think they are fattening. Some of the most popular, longstanding programs on the market such as the Atkins diet are based on the premise that you must severely restrict carbohydrates to lose weight. This is not true. Because you need a basic amount of carbohydrates just to keep brain function and other metabolic processes efficient, low-carbohydrate diets can make you feel exhausted and irritable. No one can stay on a diet for long that leaves them depleted of energy and unable to concentrate.

A very low-carbohydrate diet (or fasting) can induce ketosis. This condition occurs when the body is unable to completely burn fat for energy. Ketones are by-products of the incompletely burned fat. If there is no glucose (carbohydrates) available, then the body (including the brain) can use ketones for energy. The World Health Organization recommends at least 50 grams of carbohydrates daily to avoid ketosis.

In the Fat-Burning Metabolic Fitness Nutritional Plan presented in this book, I ask readers to eat a diet that includes 40 percent low-glycemic carbohydrates. Choosing the correct kind of carbohydrates is an important part of losing weight, maintaining weight, and staying healthy. Sugary and overprocessed foods such as candy, cake, and soft drinks are simple carbohydrates. Bran muffins, brown rice, and whole-grain breads are complex carbohydrates. Also, each fruit, vegetable, and grain has a different rate of digestion based on the glycemic index. Carbohydrates that digest slowly and release their energy into the bloodstream gradually result in less stored fat than those that digest quickly, releasing their energy in amounts greater than the body can use.

Fear of Fats

Many people are afraid of eating fats because they associate them with instant weight gain. When my nutritionist, Molly Kimball, evaluates clients for my health and performance enhancement program (PEP), she often finds that people who are trying to lose weight frequently avoid fats. They believe that everything they eat must be low-fat or fat-free. This makes for a boring and tasteless diet. Their typical breakfast might be dry toast or a bagel or cereal with low-fat milk. Lunch might be a sandwich with very little meat and no mayonnaise or cheese. Dinner might be pasta, brown rice, or a potato and with a little protein. Eating all of these carbohydrates by themselves without a sufficient amount of lean meat (30 percent of the total diet) and acceptable fats (30 percent of the total diet) can trigger an insulin release, causing blood sugar to dip.

No one can avoid fats and stay healthy. Because fat is an energy source, your body needs a certain amount to function efficiently. Most fats are commonly found in animal foods or can be synthesized in your body from carbohydrates. However, your body cannot make these essential fatty acids, which are omega-6 and omega-3. A deficiency of essential fatty acids will produce symptoms such as dry and scaly skin, dermatitis, and hair loss.

Clients are often shocked to find out how the pounds begin to drop when they begin eating the right amount of fats. Again, the type of fats that you eat—mono- and polyunsaturated fats versus saturated fats—is the most important factor in weight loss, weight maintenance, and good health.

Studies have shown that a healthy nutritional program consists of 40 percent low-glycemic carbohydrates, 30 percent lean protein, and 30 percent acceptable fats.

Fact #4: Controlling Your Insulin Response Is Key for Fat Loss

The most effective way to reduce body fat and promote metabolic efficiency is to normalize your body's ability to manage insulin. Effectively managing insulin is based on four factors: (1) the glycemic index of the foods you eat (their complexity and the amount of time it takes to digest them), (2) the efficiency of your metabolism, (3) your fat–to–lean muscle ratio, and (4) the amount and type of physical activity and exercise you engage in.

Since muscle tissue is metabolically active and fat just basically sits there, the fatter you are, the less metabolically active your body will be. There are two main scenarios in which a person develops a high fat–to–lean muscle ratio. The first can occur at any age and is lifestyle related—high levels of stress, poor eating habits, low levels of exercise or no exercise. The second is a natural but reversible process called sarcopenia that develops with age. Sarcopenia is basically the wasting of lean muscle and the gain in body fat that results from lack of exercise, especially resistive exercise. Whatever the reason, having an unhealthy amount of body fat can lead to a lower metabolic rate and insulin resistance.

Insulin is the hormone involved in storing energy from the foods that we eat. When there is an overabundance of energy-giving foods in a meal, especially carbohydrates but to a lesser degree proteins and to a much lesser degree fats, the body will secrete insulin in great quantities. Any nutrients that cannot be used at that time will be stored. Insulin affects excess proteins by promoting amino acid uptake by cells. Insulin causes excess carbohydrates to be stored as glycogen in the liver, muscles, and circulatory system until they are needed between meals when glucose levels drop. All of the excess carbohydrates that cannot be stored as glycogen are converted into fat and stored in the adipose (fatty) tissues.

The book *Endocrinology and Reproduction* by P. C. K. Leung and others gives further insights into this process in the chapter where it discusses insulin and diabetes: "When insulin is secreted into the blood, it circulates almost entirely in an unbound form: it has a plasma half-life that averages only about 6 minutes, so that it is mainly cleared from the circulation within 10 to 15 minutes. . . . This rapid removal from the plasma is important because at times it is equally as important to turn off rapidly as to turn on the control functions of insulin."

When a person becomes overfat, especially in the abdominal area, he or she can become insulin resistant. Muscle cells, which make up 30 to 50 percent of the body, get out of shape and lose much of their ability to respond effectively to insulin. This leaves a surplus of glucose floating around in the blood—much more than the body actually needs for its immediate energy needs. In turn, the pancreas is stimulated to release even more insulin to do its job of transporting the glucose through the cell membranes.

Since the fat cells of an overfat individual are more receptive to insulin than the muscle cells, this is where much of the remaining glucose eventually gets deposited. A vicious cycle is created, causing even more fat gain—that is, the more overfat a person becomes, the more excess carbohydrates will be converted into fat storage.

Most people did not become overfat during the centuries of hunting and farming, primarily because our ancestors ate more complex foods and engaged in more physical work, which caused a more stable insulin response and resulted in leaner, stronger, healthier bodies. These complex foods, which take longer to digest, included whole grains, legumes, and vegetables, all of which have a high fiber content and are low in simple sugars.

The glycemic index rates foods according to the speed at which they are digested and converted to energy or stored. Foods with a low glycemic index are more complex and require burning more calories to digest them. Foods with a high glycemic index digest quickly; therefore, if they are not burned during daily activities, they are usually stored as fat because your body is genetically programmed to store the food energy that you cannot use immediately. This goes back to the feast-or-famine idea discussed earlier. Since our ancestors could not always get regular meals, their bodies developed the ability to slow their metabolism and store all excess foods as fat for the lean times.

Fact #5: You Must Be Physically Active to Have an Efficient Metabolism

Metabolic efficiency is directly related to the amount of activity you engage in each day. This includes everything from planned exercise to walking through your local mall to playing with your kids to taking your spouse out dancing or your family for a walk in the local park. If you aren't physically active, you will begin to gain weight. It's that simple.

According to a recent report by the surgeon general, a shocking 60 percent of Americans do not engage in enough activity to keep them even minimally healthy, and 25 percent get no exercise at all. Many people think that metabolism slows as you get older. It is not your metabolic processes that are slowing down, however; it is your lifestyle and level of activity.

When most baby boomers think back to how they looked in their childhood, they probably remember a skinny boy or girl who was always outside running around or playing sports. When they got older and took on adult responsibilities, they may have sat behind a desk for eight hours a day. As time passed, children were born, family responsibilities increased, and they got older, they probably spent more time working and less time being physically active, resulting in gradual yearly weight gain. With the advent of television and home computers, even leisure time took on a sedentary nature, with the average adult watching four hours of TV daily. The commercials for junk food, sugary treats, soft drinks, chips, and highly processed foods also encourage poor eating habits. When was the last time you saw a TV ad for fresh fruits and vegetables?

A certain amount of inactivity is directly related to the fact that more than 50 percent of all Americans are now living in urban environments where being active outdoors is not necessarily a part of daily life. If you live in a condo or an apartment, you probably don't mow the lawn or do yard work; nor are your kids easily able to step outside and play or take a dip in the pool.

To create metabolic efficiency, you need to engage in at least twenty to thirty minutes of exercise at least three times per week. How you should exercise is related to your gender. Studies have shown that women tend to metabolize more fat at low to moderate intensities of exercise and men at moderate to high intensities. Also, as individuals get older, the ratio between aerobic and resistance exercise should change. The older a person gets, the more he or she will need to conserve bone mass and lean muscle, both of which decrease with age. The average cardiovascular and resistance exercise percentages for a person in good health with normal weight should be as follows:

Age	Cardio (%)	Resistance (%)
Under 40	70	30
40–49	40	60
50–59	50	50
60–69	40	60
70 and older	30	70

In this book I show you how to maximize the fat loss and metabolic benefits you derive from exercise.

Fact #6: Your Metabolism Loves Consistency

The one thing that your metabolic processes love the most is consistency. If you spend one month never exercising, one week overexercising, and another month exercising only occasionally, your body will not be able to get the full benefit of a consistent activity level and the benefits of a metabolism that is more efficient at fat burning. When you are constantly alternating overeating with undereating, your blood sugar and insulin response are yo-yoing up and down as your body desperately tries to figure out whether there is a feast or a famine. Eating three healthy meals per day plus two or three snacks will create maximum metabolic efficiency.

Fat-Burning Metabolic Fitness Questionnaire

This simple questionnaire should help you to understand how metabolically fit you are. If you answer no to all of the questions, you most likely have an efficient metabolism. If you answer yes to three questions, your metabolism is probably only moderately efficient and you would benefit from changing your eating and exercise patterns. If you check off more than three yes answers, your metabolism has probably slowed to the point where you are overfat. Besides changing your eating and exercise patterns, you should consider having a resting metabolic test performed by your physician, especially if you also checked off a significant number of items in the Signs and Symptoms of Hypothyroidism questionnaire in chapter 6.

Fat-Burning Metabolic Fitness Questionnaire

	Yes	No
1. Do you go for more than 3½–4 hours without eating?	☐	☐
2. Do you have an excessive buildup of abdominal fat (35 inches for a woman and 40 inches for a man)?	☐	☐
3. Have you noticed an increase in your waist circumference without a significant change in your weight?	☐	☐
4. Do you feel tired much of the time, especially midmorning and midafternoon?	☐	☐

5. Do you exercise regularly but still find that you are
   gaining fat weight?   ☐ ☐
6. Do you feel cold throughout the year?   ☐ ☐
7. If you are a woman, do you have excessive facial hair? ☐ ☐
8. Do you gain weight easily?   ☐ ☐

Total # of Yes's____ Total # of No's____

It's never too late to increase your level of metabolic fitness. Since lean muscle tissue is metabolically more active than fat, which basically just sits there, the key is to reduce fat and increase lean muscle. Regardless of your score on the Fat-Burning Metabolic Fitness Questionnaire, the metabolic prescription presented in this book will help you to bring your metabolism up to maximum efficiency.

3

Classic Female and Male Fat Patterns

The Classic Female Fat Pattern

There are many nicknames for female fat. We downplay it by using cute or nonoffensive labels such as saddlebags, chunky body, looking healthy, or dimples in the hips and thighs. Or we try to tame it, cover it up, or hold it in using a whole range of garments from girdles to control-top panty hose to baggy clothing. Entire cosmetic industries have arisen to help women get rid of unsightly cellulite and stretch marks, while attractive women's fashions in large sizes are making their mark in stores and in fashion magazines designed for those with a "generous" figure. Most women wage a lifetime battle with fat, as can be seen by the hundreds of diet books for women that fill bookstore shelves. In fact, at any given time, three out of four women are either trying to lose weight or keep it off.

While I would agree with the self-help authors who tell female readers that the key to self-esteem is to love your body, I believe that a woman should find a balance between accepting her body just as it is and paying serious attention to the significant health risks of being overfat. There is nothing life-affirming about having type 2 diabetes, painful and over-stressed joints, and an increased risk of heart disease after menopause. As we have seen, being overfat also increases the risk of certain types of cancers. For example, a recent report published by the National Cancer Institute showed that women with a Body Mass Index (BMI) of 30 or greater were twice as likely to develop cervical cancer. Women with the lowest waist-to-hip ratio, indicating a significant accumulation of abdominal fat, were eight times more likely to develop this disease than women with a normal waist-to-hip ratio.

To better understand how a woman's body fat can become a risk for her, let's take a look at the physiological and hormonal processes involved in female fat storage.

The Importance of the Body Fat–to–Lean Muscle Ratio

Even though most women equate being overfat with how many pounds they weigh, the scale does not tell the whole story. While scale weight is certainly an important factor and will give you some information about your general health, it is even more important for you to determine your body composition—that is, how many pounds of fat you carry in relationship to how many pounds of lean muscle. The following table categorizes body fat percentages for women:

Body Fat (%)	Level
<14	Athletic
14–17	Good/lean
18–22	Average
23–27	Fair/fat
27+	Obese

If you compare these figures with the body fat percentages of men, you will see that healthy women tend to carry approximately 10 percent more body fat. This is nature's way of giving women a small and much-needed fuel surplus for pregnancy, breast-feeding, and child rearing.

Most women believe that it is inevitable that their body fat–to–lean muscle ratio will rise as they age and experience the hormonal changes associated with menopause. In fact, the tables you see in some health books, on the Internet, or in your doctor's office will reflect this belief, allowing for a higher "healthy" percentage of body fat in older people. But women do not have to settle for a higher fat percentage as they reach midlife and their later years. The amount of body fat is directly related to diet, exercise, lifestyle, and hormonal balance.

While it's unlikely that a seventy-year-old woman is going to have 14 percent body fat, she shouldn't be content to settle for an unhealthy amount of fat. It is never too late to improve your body composition through a good nutritional and exercise program. And, I might add, it's never too early. In recent years in my Fat-Burning Metabolic Fitness Plan, I have been seeing women in their twenties and thirties with a high percentage of body fat. One thirty-eight-year-old female client who is 5 feet 8 inches and weighed 158 pounds didn't really consider herself to have a weight problem until we tested her and she saw that her body fat was 34.5 percent, which made her technically obese.

In contrast, since I work with many world-class female athletes, I often see clients whose larger, more muscular bodies cause them to weigh more than the average woman of their height and frame size. In their case, however, they have a very low percentage of body fat and a higher-than-average percentage of lean muscle. A good example would be a female body builder or a competitor in any type of sport where strength is required.

Chapter 4 has a simple at-home test to measure your body fat–to–lean muscle ratio.

The Classic Female Body Type

By now it should be clear that the most important issue is not just how fat you are but if your level of body fat is within the healthy range. Where do you carry your fat and when does fat become a problem?

The classic female body type is the gynoid shape—that is, fat storage below the waist in the hip and buttocks areas, causing a pear-shaped silhouette. Since weight below the waist presents less of a health risk than abdominal fat, an overweight woman actually has a lower risk than an overweight man for certain illnesses such as heart disease. An article in the *British Medical Journal* states, "Recent studies have also shown that a preferential accumulation of body fat in the glutofemoral region [hips and thighs], commonly found in premenopausal women and initially described by Vague [a French physician] under the term 'gynoid obesity' is not a major threat to cardiovascular health."

Learn the Dangers of the Reverse Fat Pattern

All bets are off, however, when a woman begins to develop what I have described as a reverse fat pattern—that is, fat in the abdominal region. Although many people think of cardiovascular disease as a man's disease, it kills more than half a million women per year. It just affects women ten to fifteen years later than the average high-risk male. A woman's risk for heart attack gradually increases following menopause precisely because that is the time when she is most likely to be storing excess fat in the abdominal region. One of the reasons is that her body is producing less of the hormone estrogen, which has a positive effect on fat mobilization.

Even though women have their first heart attacks later than men, they are more likely to die from them. Within one year of having an attack, 25 percent of men die, but 38 percent of women die. According to a recent article in *Health Day News,* women are also more likely than men to be physically disabled by a stroke and/or to have speech difficulties, visual impairment, and difficulty chewing and swallowing. On average, women's hospital stays were longer by three days. These are all good motivations to lose that excess abdominal fat.

Women are also less likely to experience the traditional chest pains that warn of heart problems in men. Instead they will complain of abdominal discomfort, nausea, vomiting, fatigue, and shortness of breath. The American Heart Association warns that even though heart attacks are more likely to kill women after they turn sixty-five because they have lost much of the protective value of estrogen and other hormones, coronary events kill 20,000 younger women each year because they do not recognize the gender-specific symptoms of heart problems. Of course, the more obese a younger woman is and the more weight she carries in her abdominal area, the more at risk she will be.

A woman with a reverse fat pattern, whatever her age might be, is also at greater risk for developing type 2 diabetes; certain types of cancer; problems with weight-supporting joints in her hips, knees, and ankles; and foot problems because of the greater constrictive design of women's footwear.

In my Fat-Burning Metabolic Fitness Plan, I work with many women who have a reverse fat pattern caused by being overfat. Many of them suffer from significant hormonal imbalances. The primary hormones affected are estrogen, testosterone, progesterone, and human growth hormone (HGH). A significant number of these morbidly obese women also experience the symptoms of hypothyroidism.

Cushing's Syndrome

In rare cases the appearance of the reverse fat pattern in women can be caused by Cushing's syndrome. Dr. Richard Milani, the vice chairperson of the Department of Cardiology at the Ochsner Heart and Vascular Institute, New Orleans, Louisiana, says that Cushing's syndrome is a relatively rare hormonal disorder caused by prolonged exposure to high levels of cortisol, a hormone produced by the adrenal gland. It usually results in abdominal obesity with sparing (thin or slender) of the arms and legs. There is often rounding of the face and thickening of the fat pads around the neck. Additionally, there are pronounced pink-purple stretch marks as well as thin and fragile skin. Women usually have excess hair growth on their face, chest, abdomen, and thighs. Irritability, anxiety, and depression are common. There are various causes of excess cortisol production including tumors that secrete or stimulate cortisol production. Cushing's syndrome can also be caused by prolonged use of high doses of prednisone. This condition can be evaluated by blood tests, and treatment is based on the cause in a given individual.

Further Dangers of Abdominal Fat: Metabolic Syndrome X

Overfat women often exhibit one or more of a whole cluster of symptoms that doctors call Metabolic Syndrome X. These include a waist circumference of 35 inches or more, triglycerides greater than 150 mg/dl, HDL (good cholesterol) less than 50 mg/dl, a fasting glucose greater than 110 mg/dl, and blood pressure greater than 135/85 mm/Hg. Anyone who has three or more of these symptoms is diagnosed with metabolic syndrome X. In chapter 4, I include a questionnaire to help you determine whether you have this syndrome. It is important because this combination of symptoms can be a strong indicator that you are at risk within the next ten years for a major cardiovascular event such as heart disease.

The Pros and Cons of the Waist-to-Hip Ratio

Since women naturally store excess fat in the hips and thighs, traditionally one of the best indicators of whether you are overfat is your waist-to-hip ratio. In chapter 4, I show you how to accurately measure your waist-to-hip ratio. I have found, however, that when a woman begins to exhibit a reverse fat pattern with abdominal fat, this measurement can often become inaccurate.

In a recent article published in the *British Medical Journal,* Dr. Jean-Pierre Despres of the Quebec Heart Institute pointed out the weakness of the waist-to hip ratio as a reliable indicator of risk for disease in women who have adopted a male fat pattern. Such individuals tend to keep gaining fat equally in the waist and the hips while their ratio remains within the "safe" range. His conclusions were based on a twenty-year study that found that once a woman begins gaining weight above the waist, her waist-to-hip ratio is no longer an accurate determination of how much body fat she is carrying: "Simultaneous increase in waist and hip measurements means ratio is stable over time despite considerable accumulation of visceral adipose tissue. . . . Thus, waist circumference provides crude index of absolute amount of abdominal adipose tissue whereas waist:hip ratio provides index of relative accumulation of abdominal fat."

For this reason, even though the waist circumference has been considered the gold standard for predicting obesity in men and the waist-to-hip ratio the gold standard for women, the waist circumference is a vitally important evaluation tool for both genders. A waist circumference of 35 inches or more spells trouble for women.

The *British Medical Journal* article also points out that when a woman experiences the reverse fat pattern, especially before menopause, it can indicate that she is a candidate for hypertriglyceridemia, which indicates an increase in the level of triglycerides in the blood, again increasing her risk for cardiovascular disease.

Gender Differences in Fat Mobilization

A cell receptor can be thought of as the parking space in which a hormone sits and does its work of turning cell function off and on. The two main types of cell receptors where epinephrine, a fat-mobilizing hormone, can "park" and act on the cell are called alpha receptors, which inhibit the breakdown of triglycerides (a.k.a. the storing of fat), and beta receptors, which stimulate the burning of fat.

Research has shown that both men and women have more beta receptors in the abdominal area, meaning that fat is easier to lose in that part of the body. But women have more alpha receptors in the hip and thigh areas than men, which explains why they tend to store more fat in those areas and why it is harder for them to lose fat.

Another factor contributing to gender differences in fat storage may be the concentration of lipoprotein lipase (LPL) in various tissues. LPL, which also regulates the mobilization of free fatty acids, is located in the walls of blood vessels throughout the body. Women have a greater concentration of LPL in the hips and thighs and a smaller concentration in the abdominal area than men.

The female hormone estrogen may have a positive effect on fat mobilization because it inhibits the fat-storing action of LPL, enhances the production of the fat-mobilizing hormone epinephrine, and stimulates the production of human growth hormone (HGH), which inhibits the storage of excess glucose by the body's tissues and increases the mobilization of free fatty acids from adipose tissue.

Kim Cummins: Watching the Inches Melt Off

I was scheduled to do three makeovers for an article in *Let's Live* magazine and was looking for people willing to undergo my twelve-week Fat-Burning Metabolic Fitness Plan. One day at lunch while I was watching my executive assistant, Kim Cummins, having a margarita, fried soft-shell crabs, and ice cream, I was suddenly hit with the inspiration that she would be the perfect candidate. When Kim had come to work for me five years earlier, she weighed 140 pounds, but since then she had gained 36 pounds, mostly because of lifestyle choices such as eating a lot of fried foods and fast foods. The joke when we went out for a meal together with clients or athletes was always "Don't eat the way Kim does; eat the way Mackie does," and "See, Kim's eating the disaster meal, but I want *you* to eat the Mackie Meal."

Kim would always laugh at me because she was young (she had just turned thirty) and felt that she could get away with anything without it adversely affecting her health. Kim ate whatever she pleased and never exercised. I remember a couple of years ago when we both had our resting metabolism tested. Kim teased me because hers was greater than mine: "See, my metabolism is a better fat burner than yours." I said, "But Kim, my body fat is 6 percent. You can joke around now, but someday in the future your lifestyle is going to come back to haunt you."

Sure enough, when my doctor gave her a health evaluation at the start of my Fat-Burning Metabolic Fitness Plan, she had some unpleasant surprises. Her body fat was 35.1 percent, her LDL (bad cholesterol) was high at 154.2 (ideally it should be between 100 and 129), and her waistline was 36 inches (remember, anything above 35 represents significant health risks). Kim knew that abdominal fat was a big strike against her. Most alarming was her C-reactive protein, which was 6.56 (the normal range is between 0 and 0.3). C-reactive protein at this level is an indicator of inflammation, which points toward a greater risk of heart attack. "My blood work was my wake-up call," she told me. "I was only *thinking* of doing the program before this. I thought it would be fun to work with a trainer and look good in my swimsuit when I went to Miami for my vacation. But the results of the blood work really decided me."

Kim never ate breakfast but ate a large lunch and dinner. It was a bit of a challenge for my nutritionist to get her on the Fat-Burning Metabolic Fitness Nutritional Plan with enough fiber because she did not like vegetables and hated breakfast foods. Kim said, "If you can make spinach taste like ice cream, I'll eat it. Otherwise, forget it." I told her that if she would learn to eat fiber-rich vegetables, she would see a rapid decrease in her body fat. She even agreed to go to a hypnotist to see if she could overcome her aversion to vegetables, but to no avail.

In spite of this obstacle, we managed to find a food plan with which Kim felt comfortable, and she began eating three large meals and two snacks a day. At first it was a challenge for her to eat all that food, but she was so determined to follow the plan that she actually set an alarm clock to remind her to stop work and grab a snack. She knew it was important for her to eat at least every four hours to boost and stabilize her metabolism.

Within a very short time, Kim noticed a dramatic change in her energy. She told me, "My energy increased unbelievably. Food had never been an obsession with me. My problem was that I didn't eat often enough. Come afternoon, I'd be so tired that one time I actually fell asleep at the wheel of my car at a red light. It was only for a second, but it totally freaked me out. I knew if I'd taken my foot off my brake I would have hit the person in front of me." But now she never feels that afternoon slump. Her sleep has also become more restful. Even though she'd always been a heavy sleeper who had trouble getting out of bed in the morning, Kim told me that she was waking up filled with energy before her alarm clock went off.

We took photos at the beginning of the Fat-Burning Metabolic Fitness Plan, then at one-month intervals. A second turning point came for Kim when she compared her before picture with her after picture at one month. Kim told me that she really wasn't expecting much after only thirty days. She'd noticed that her muscles were getting harder, especially her legs, which had never been muscular before, and that she was losing inches, but she'd only lost 5 pounds of scale weight. I told her not to worry because I could see that she was losing fat and gaining lean muscle.

When Kim actually compared the two pictures, she burst into tears. "I didn't realize how fat my face had become. You always lose weight in the last place you put it on. My face had gone from being round and fat to real slender and skinny. I just couldn't believe how big it had been and how much of a difference there was now. I was only expecting small changes in the second photo. When I saw the results, I realized that I had been expecting that much change at the end of three months. It was a dramatic difference after only one month. I was in shock."

At the end of three months, Kim was feeling great. Her statistics demonstrate the changes her body went through:

Measure	Start	End
Waistline	36 in.	32.75 in. (a loss of 3.25 in.)
Hip	43 in.	41 in. (a loss of 2 in.)
BMI	25.46	24.11 (a drop of 1.35 points into the lower-risk range)
C-reactive protein	6.56	3.73 (a drop of 2.83 points)
Total cholesterol	223	209 (a drop of 14 points)
LDL	154.2	130 (a drop of 24.2 points)
HDL	50	50 (still within the healthiest range for women)
Lipoprotein a	20	11 (a loss of 9 points)

Although she had only lost 10 pounds of scale weight at that point, she had lost much more than that in actual pounds of body fat. I often see this in clients—a kind of conversion process where the fat melts off and they lose inches all over their body as they replace it with lean muscle. When we measured Kim's fat–to–lean muscle ratio, she had 22 pounds of fat and 144 pounds of lean muscle, which made her very happy. She told me that she looked so slimmed down that everyone thought she'd lost about 50 pounds.

Kim is indicative of many young women who fall into the trap of eating poorly, who give up exercise in favor of working long hours at a career they enjoy, and who start experiencing a metabolic slowdown with its accompanying gradual accumulation of body fat at an early age. These lifestyle choices are a one-way ticket to disaster.

To this day, Kim continues to follow the Fat-Burning Metabolic Fitness Plan because it has made such a difference in her life. She feels better than she's felt in years and looks great. Most important, she's stopped a trend in body fat gain that would have greatly lessened the quality of her life as she reached middle age and quite probably might have resulted in serious illness later on and a much shorter life span.

The Classic Male Fat Pattern

Fat in men has been christened with a variety of names. We call it the beer belly, the spare tire, or simply the gut. We joke about it, calling it Dunlap's disease ("His stomach done lapped over his belt") or give it a playful label such as love handles. But there is nothing humorous about abdominal fat. It is a dangerous health risk that can lead to complications such as cardiovascular disease, some types of cancer, hypertension, type 2 diabetes, and erectile dysfunction.

To better understand the dangers of abdominal fat, let's take a look at what body processes are involved in male fat storage.

The Importance of the Body Fat–to–Lean Muscle Ratio

When most people think about how fat or thin they are, they think about how many scale pounds they weigh. While your weight on the scale is certainly important and will give you some information about your general health, it is even more important for you to determine your body composition—that is, how many pounds of fat you carry in relationship to how many pounds of lean muscle. The following table categorizes body fat percentages for men:

Body Fat (%)	Level
<11	Athletic
11–14 percent	Good/lean
15–17 percent	Average
18–22 percent	Fair/fat
22+ percent	Obese

Most men believe that it is inevitable that their body fat–to–lean muscle ratio will rise as they age and experience the hormonal changes associated with andropause. In fact, the tables you see in some health books, on the Internet, or in your doctor's office will reflect this belief, allowing for a higher "healthy" percentage of body fat in older people. But men do not have to settle for a higher fat percentage as they reach midlife and their later years. The amount of body fat is directly related to diet and exercise.

While it's unlikely that a seventy-year-old man is going to have 11 percent body fat, he shouldn't be content to settle for an unhealthy amount of fat. It is never too late to change your body composition through a good nutritional and exercise program. And, I might add, it's never too early. I have seen men in their twenties and thirties with high percentages of body fat, especially in sports such as football where large size is important. Chapter 4 has an at-home test to measure your body fat–to–lean muscle ratio.

Scale Weight Does Not Tell the Whole Story about Fat

If your percentage of fat versus lean muscle is the true indicator of whether you have a healthy body composition, then how much you weigh on the scale does not really give you an accurate idea of how overfat you may be. Let's look at two athletes who weigh 240 pounds.

The first man, Jon, is a body builder with 10 percent body fat; all the rest is lean muscle. Jon's metabolism is very efficient because lean muscle is metabolically very active. His appearance is firm and muscular, his waistline is trim, and his abdomen is flat. His general health is excellent, his lipid profile (triglycerides and cholesterol) is well within the normal range, and he feels energized and alert throughout the day.

The second man, Paul, has 40 percent body fat and looks and feels completely different. Even though he is an NFL lineman, his metabolism is not as efficient as it should be because body fat is not metabolically active. His body looks overfat, his waistline measures 48 inches, and his stomach bulges over his belt. His cholesterol and triglyceride levels are dangerously high. Because he carries so much weight in the abdominal area, he is seriously at risk for type 2 diabetes and cardiovascular disease (if he doesn't already suffer from these diseases not yet diagnosed). Even though he is a professional athlete, his body does not feel fit and his heavy stomach puts a strain on his lower back. He often complains of back, knee, and hip pain from all of the extra fat he drags around.

Where Do You Carry Your Weight?

By now it should be clear that the most important issue is not just how fat you are but where you carry your fat and the point at which it becomes a problem.

The classic male fat pattern is the apple or android shape—weight above the waist. Therefore, the waist measurement in a man is one of the most accurate indicators of how much at risk he is for a variety of serious diseases. In 2002, when the American Heart Association published their revised "Guide to the Primary Prevention of Cardiovascular Diseases" in *Circulation* magazine, they warned that a waist measurement of 40 inches or more in a man indicated a greater chance of developing cardiovascular disease. Dr. Sidney C. Smith, the association's chief science officer, was quoted as saying, "It's turned out that waist circumference is as good a predictor of risk as body mass index."

In my Fat-Burning Metabolic Fitness Plan, I have found that waist circumference is a better indicator of health risks than BMI. For example, the waistline measurement is an especially good tool in evaluating older men who have not gained weight but have undergone unhealthy changes in body composition. I have seen many clients in their sixties and seventies whose weight has not gone up in years—that is, their BMI has not changed—but they have gained inches in the waistline, indicating a loss of lean muscle and an increase in body fat. Some people swear by the waist-to-hip ratio as a good evaluation tool, but I always look primarily at the waist measurement in men, because when a man has a reverse fat pattern, his waist-to-hip ratio can remain constant over time while he is actually storing quite a bit of fat in that part of the body.

Vulnerability to certain diseases can even be present in a man whose waistline is less than 40 inches. Depending on how clients measure up during their initial health evaluation and how much body fat–to–lean muscle they have, my doctors usually suggest that some men take a glucose tolerance test or a hemoglobin A1C test, which follows a person's blood sugar over a two- to three-month period if his waistline has reached 37 inches. This is because there is such a high correlation between excess abdominal fat and insulin resistance, a precursor to type 2 diabetes.

I have also seen a direct correlation between erectile dysfunction and abdominal fat. A 2000 study funded by the National Cancer Institute found that men with a waistline measurement of 42 inches or more were twice as likely to suffer from erectile dysfunction than men with a waistline measuring 32 inches. Men who were inactive were also more prone to this problem than men who exercised at least thirty minutes a day.

This information was confirmed by the results of a 2003 study of nearly 32,000 men aged 53 to 90 reported in the *Annals of Internal Medicine*. Researchers found that one out of three older men suffered from erectile dysfunction. However, men who were not overfat and who exercised regularly were 30 percent less likely to have this condition.

Further Dangers of Abdominal Fat: Metabolic Syndrome X

Overfat men often exhibit one or more of a whole cluster of symptoms that doctors call Metabolic Syndrome X. These include a waistline of 40 inches or more, triglycerides greater than 150 mg/dl, HDL (good cholesterol) less than 40 mg/dl, a fasting glucose greater than 110 mg/dl, and blood pressure greater than 135/85 mm/Hg. Anyone who has three or more of these symptoms is diagnosed with Metabolic Syndrome X. In chapter 4, I include a questionnaire to help you determine whether you have this syndrome. It is important because this combination of symptoms can be a strong indicator that you are at risk within the next ten years for a major cardiovascular event such as heart disease.

In a recent article published in the *British Medical Journal,* Dr. Jean-Pierre Despres of the Quebec Heart Institute referred to Metabolic Syndrome X as hypertriglyceridemia and confirmed the risk for heart disease that the symptoms above represented when coupled with a waistline of over 40 inches. Dr. Despres also pointed out the weakness of the waist-to-hip ratio as a reliable indicator of risk for disease, since men who had adopted a female fat pattern tended to keep gaining fat in the waist and hips while their ratio remained within the "safe" range.

Don't Be Defeated by the "Beer Belly Gene"

I have heard many men make the excuse that they carry abdominal fat because of their DNA. Every man in their family has a huge gut and therefore they themselves are doomed to this "genetic" condition of being overfat.

In most instances, I have discovered that this is not the case. Overfat individuals almost always grow up in—and continue to live in—an environment where their family, friends, and loved ones all have poor eating and exercising habits. They are obese because of their lifestyle and unhealthy nutrition habits, not because of some mysterious fat gene.

However, in a minority of men, scientists have found something that they have dubbed the "beer belly gene." A recent study conducted by a team of researchers at the University of Naples and published in the *Annals of Internal Medicine* found that of 959 men between the ages of twenty-five and seventy-five, a small percentage did have a genetic variation that predisposed them to develop abdominal fat.

This genetic predisposition does not spell doom, however. The bottom line was that these men had a greater *propensity* to develop an unhealthy amount of abdominal fat *if and only if* they led an unhealthy lifestyle. None of these men got beer guts from eating nutritious foods and exercising regularly. And they had just as much chance of losing fat and increasing their lean muscle mass as men without the beer belly gene. In the case of these men, if they wanted to keep the fat off, they would just have to be a bit more vigilant in their lifestyle.

Learn Why Exercising Increases Fat Loss

We've seen the many health risks associated with abdominal fat. Now for the good news: *abdominal fat is the easiest type of body fat to lose.*

Fat is stored in cells in the form of triglycerides. You've heard that exercise increases the body's ability to burn fat, but probably you've never really understood why that happens—or, for that matter, why you should even bother to exercise if you're already on a good food program. Shouldn't just eating correctly be enough? In reality, appropriate exercise greatly enhances your body's ability to burn stored fat.

Epinephrine is a fat-mobilizing hormone released by your sympathetic nervous system. Studies have shown that during exercise there is a significantly greater concentration of this hormone in your body. When epinephrine binds to specific receptors on fat cells, it stimulates hormone-sensitive lipase, also known as HSL, to break apart triglycerides within the cells and release them into the bloodstream where they can be used as energy. And that's precisely what you want to happen. You don't want that fat to just sit around in your body; you want to get it mobilized.

When you engage in aerobic exercise, HSL becomes even more sensitive to epinephrine since your body temperature is rising. The greater your aerobic endurance, the less concentration of epinephrine it will take to activate HSL and release stored fat. If you are obese, however, it will take significantly higher amounts of this hormone to stimulate the breakdown of triglycerides.

Another hormone affected by exercise is leptin, a peptide hormone produced by the adipose (fatty) tissue that plays a role in the storing of body fat and in overall energy balance. A recent study published in the *Journal of Nutritional Biochemistry* states that exercise combined with dieting is the most effective combination to reduce levels of leptin in the body, with a resulting loss of body fat.

The Secret to Abdominal Fat Loss: Alpha Receptors and Beta Receptors

A cell receptor can be thought of as the parking space in which a hormone sits and does its work of turning cell function off and on. The two main types of cell receptors where epinephrine, a fat-mobilizing hormone, can "park" and act on the cell are called alpha receptors, which inhibit the breakdown of triglycerides (a.k.a. the storing of fat), and beta receptors, which stimulate the burning of fat.

Research has shown that both men and women have more beta receptors in the abdominal area, meaning that fat is easier to lose in that part of the body. But women have more alpha receptors in the hip and thigh areas than men, which explains why they tend to store more fat in those areas.

The core body exercises in this book are specifically designed to enable your body to mobilize its fat-burning capacity to reduce the abdominal area of your body.

Dangers of the Reverse Fat Pattern

The most unhealthy areas in which a man can gain fat are in the hips and buttocks. This is known as the reverse fat pattern, because it mimics the classic areas where women most often gain weight. By the time a man has crossed over into a reverse fat pattern, his waistline usually measures 50 inches or more and he is considered to be morbidly obese. As already stated, it is much more difficult for a man to mobilize fat in this part of the body than it is in the abdominal region.

I work with many men who have a reverse fat pattern. Many of them suffer from significant hormonal imbalances. They exhibit low testosterone, higher than normal levels of estradiol (which is the primary hormone in females), lower sex drive, erectile dysfunction, and low thyroid. The lowered testosterone and higher estradiol levels often result in gynecomastia, in which a man's breasts become soft and prominent like a woman's. As a man's body becomes "feminized" by excess fat, he has a much lower than average percentage of lean muscle and suffers from decreased strength, irritability, and chronic exhaustion.

Success in Combating the Reverse Male Fat Pattern

Douglas Daniels, a forty-one-year-old New Orleans French Quarter nightclub performer, was a classic example of the reverse fat pattern. When Douglas first entered my Fat-Burning Metabolic Fitness Plan to be evaluated, he was so morbidly obese that our doctors gave him five years maximum to live. Here are his health statistics before beginning my plan:

Height	5'8"
Weight	368 lb.
Cholesterol	201
Triglycerides	567
Glucose	283
Waist	61 in.
Hips	66 in.
BMI	57.88

Notice that Douglas's hips are 5 inches larger than his waist, indicating a reverse fat pattern where he not only carries fat in his abdomen but in his hips and buttocks.

Douglas was a two-pack-a-day smoker, increasing his potential risk of heart disease and cancer, and he suffered from sleep apnea, a disease that can damage the heart if left untreated. He had to take an oral medication called glucophage for type 2 diabetes. He suffered from low testosterone and hypothyroidism. He was a walking time bomb, and I knew that I had to motivate him to save his own life—fast.

Our doctor immediately put him on thyroid medication and enrolled him in our Ochsner Cardiac Rehabilitation Program, where he worked to increase his aerobic fitness. During that time he did resistance exercises with light dumbbells and exercises to strengthen and stabilize the core area of his body. One of the most important steps was to dramatically overhaul his nutritional regimen, which then consisted of large amounts of fatty fried foods and rich, high-calorie pasta dishes that his mother and his fiancée cooked for him. Douglas and his girlfriend learned how to make delicious low-fat Italian dishes and healthier "N'awlins"-style meals and to enjoy the low-glycemic, low-saturated-fat Mackie Meals that nutritionist Molly Kimball and I have developed for my clients (see chapter 10).

After six weeks, Douglas continued with the food program and graduated to performing an exercise program that contained added cardio and interval training to his resistance and core exercises. I also gave him tools for reducing stress and staying motivated.

By the end of the twelve-week makeover for the Discovery Health Channel show, *Health Cops New Orleans,* Douglas's statistics had changed dramatically:

Weight	310 lb. (a loss of 58 lb.)
Cholesterol	142 (a loss of 59 points)
Triglycerides	95 (a loss of 472 points!)
Glucose	107 (a loss of 176 points)
Waist	52 in. (a loss of 9 in.)
Hips	54.5 in. (a loss of 11.5 in.)
BMI	48.75 (a drop of 9.13 points)

Douglas has quit smoking, no longer snores, and no longer has to take his medication for diabetes. He has faithfully followed the program and continues to lose weight and build lean muscle mass. Twenty weeks after he started, he had lost an additional 33 pounds, bringing him to a grand total of 91 pounds of scale weight lost!

If my Fat-Burning Metabolic Fitness Plan can work on someone who was as far gone as Douglas, you know it can work for you. If he and literally hundreds of other overfat men and women with significant health risks can turn themselves around using the plan presented in this book, what are you waiting for? There's really no excuse not to begin today.

4

Evaluate Your
Health and Fat Patterns

Usually being overfat is something that creeps up gradually with age. One of the last things my team and I always do when we evaluate people who enroll in my Fat-Burning Metabolic Fitness Plan is take front-, back-, and side-view "before" photographs so that they can really and truly see what they look like and compare these images with their "after" photos. For most, it is a great surprise to suddenly perceive an overweight person on the film because our inner image of ourselves is usually much thinner, leaner, and younger. I have had clients express shock or even burst into tears when they really looked at these pictures. It is truly as if they were seeing themselves for the first time.

While I find it important to help my clients establish an accurate perception of their outward appearance, it is also important to help them establish an accurate perception of their internal health. Knowing that you are bulging over the belt of your pants or your skirt does not tell you anything about your cholesterol, triglycerides, or percentage of body fat versus lean muscle.

Are You as Healthy as You Look?

I often work with men and women who everyone else would consider healthy because they are elite athletes at the height of their profession, and they are paid huge salaries to play their sport. A highly respected NFL lineman, 6 feet 5 inches, came into my program weighing 328 pounds. He had a BMI greater than 36, a 51.7-inch waist, and a total cholesterol of 227. His HDL was low at 29. Since his triglycerides were 467, we couldn't get an accurate reading on his LDL because, as my doctors tell me, excessively high triglycerides almost always skew the LDL reading. His glucose was 120, just 6 points below the diabetic classification. The real shocker was his blood pressure, which was 190/120. We found out that he had stopped taking his blood pressure medicine and failed to tell either his trainer or the team doctor. If he had not come to us for help, it is highly likely that in the near future he would have had a stroke right there on the field. And this man was considered to be a world-class athlete.

The appearance of health is not always the same as true health. Sometimes the way a person looks can be very deceiving, especially in the case of someone who is fairly slim and exercises regularly. I once worked with a thirty-three-year-old world champion athlete. With a body fat of 9 percent, this man was certainly not overweight. But when we evaluated him, we found that he had an abnormal stress test, an elevated total cholesterol of 260, and an LDL of 190. When we took his family history, we discovered that there was a lot of heart disease present. If this man had continued to ignore his cholesterol for ten more years, he would have ended up with damage to his arteries, resulting in cardiovascular problems.

Learn How to Accurately Evaluate Your Health

With all of the confusing information in the media and in diet and fitness books these days, people really do not have a good idea of what constitutes a healthy body. Our parents never taught us—they didn't grow up eating processed foods, living a physically inactive lifestyle, and facing the kinds of daily stressors that we face—and the great majority of us do not have wellness programs in our workplace. Nor do we understand how to monitor our health and risk factors as we grow older. Somehow we have developed the misconception that staying vigorous and healthy is an intuitive process.

That is why it is so important to have the proper tools for health evaluation. During my thirty years of experience with thousands of clients as a performance enhancement and fitness consultant, I have come to clearly understand the definitions of good health and poor health because I have seen these scenarios played out so many times. And the dozens of top medical professionals with whom I have worked in my Fat-Burning Metabolic

Fitness Plan and the Ochsner Clinic Foundation have helped to acquaint me intimately with the science behind state-of-the-art health care and health evaluation.

The Fat-Burning Metabolic Fitness Plan questionnaires presented in this book are simple and straightforward guides to help you understand how overfat you are and how healthy you really are, both inside and out. Some people will find that they might not have to lose an enormous amount of weight, but they will need to lower their cholesterol, raise their HDL, reduce their overall body fat, develop healthy eating habits, and/or learn how to exercise properly. Others will discover that they are seriously overfat and will face life-threatening health risks such as heart disease and type 2 diabetes unless they change their lifestyle.

The Fat-Burning Metabolic Fitness Self-Evaluation in this chapter covers two main areas:

1. How you measure up. This includes common indicators of risk factors such as high scale weight, body fat percentage, BMI, and waist measurement.
2. Your overall body measurements, which will help you see where you are holding your fat. These measurements will be retaken at the end of the basic four-week Fat-Burning Metabolic Fitness Plan (and every four weeks after that if you continue with Modules 2 and 3) to help you quantify how much body fat you are actually losing and how hard and lean you are becoming.

You are only as strong as your weakest link. But be assured that the lifestyle, nutritional, and exercise programs offered in this book have worked for thousands of overfat men and women.

I suggest that you make a photocopy of the Fat-Burning Metabolic Fitness Self-Evaluation Questionnaire so that you can keep a record of your progress. As you work your way through each section of this chapter, you will learn how to fill in the blanks. I describe why each of these criteria is an important indicator of overall health and how you can use them to build an accurate picture of how you measure up. In subsequent chapters I will help you to evaluate your lipid profile and glucose levels, your level of human growth hormone and your thyroid function, and your stress levels.

The Fat-Burning Metabolic Fitness
Self-Evaluation Questionnaire

Age _____
Gender _____
Height _____
Scale Weight _____ lb.
% Body Fat _____
Fat _____ lb.
Lean Muscle _____ lb.
Body Mass Index _____

Overall Body Measurements:

Arm _____ in.
Forearm _____ in.
Chest _____ in.
Waist _____ in.
Abdomen _____ in.
Hips _____ in.
Thigh _____ in.
Calf _____ in.
Waist-to-Hip Ratio _____

How Do You Measure Up?
Learn the Six Basic Health Criteria

Health Criterion #1: Scale Weight

Weight gain has become a problem of epic proportions in our society. In 1905, only 5 percent of the population was obese, but that figure has been growing at an alarming rate. In the last decade alone, obesity has risen 8 percent. About 97 million people over age twenty—that is, 60 percent—are either overweight or obese. Of that number, 12.5 million are severely overweight, and 2 million are morbidly obese. These people are at great risk for life-threatening health conditions such as heart disease, stroke, diabetes, and some types of cancer.

You need to know your scale weight to complete the Fat-Burning Metabolic Fitness Self-Evaluation Questionnaire. To get an accurate scale weight that you can track over the twelve weeks of this program, it is important to have access to a fairly good scale—either a good bathroom scale or one at your gym. Ideally, you should weigh yourself nude first thing in the morning before you have eaten breakfast. If you weigh yourself with clothing at the gym or at a doctor's office, you might deduct 1 or 2 pounds for shoes and clothes.

Health Criterion #2: Body Fat

Your scale weight does not tell the whole story—far from it. A bodybuilder might weigh 250 pounds on the scale but have a total body fat of 8 percent. Someone might not be that much overweight according to the scale but may carry an unhealthy amount of body fat for his or her age. Men or women with big bones and a large frame will naturally weigh more than those with small bones and a delicate frame. To really understand how overfat you are, you need to calculate how many of your scale pounds represent body fat. This chart defines healthy and unhealthy body fat percentages for men and women:

BODY FAT PERCENTAGE

Level	Men	Women
Athletic	<11	<14
Good/lean	11–14	14–17
Average	15–17	18–22
Fair/fat	18–22	23–27
Obese	22+	27+

It used to be that men and women past age fifty were expected to be out of shape and carrying a larger amount of body fat. Some charts in doctors' offices or magazine articles will even allow greater amounts of "healthy" body fat for men and women who are middle-aged or older. I do not really follow those guidelines because experience has shown me that people in their fifties, sixties, or even seventies do not have less of a capacity to lose body fat and build lean muscle than younger people. An article in the *Canadian Journal of Applied Physiology* reports that studies on sarcopenia (loss of lean muscle mass with aging) unequivocally show that older muscle tissue has the same, if not an even greater capacity, to respond to a vigorous bout of resistance exercise than younger muscle does.

Age is not the issue; metabolic fitness is the issue—that is, how efficiently your metabolism burns fat, which is based on how much lean muscle you have, what and how often you eat, how much and at what intensity you exercise, and how balanced your body's hormonal systems are, especially those hormones that regulate the burning of nutrients as fuel or cause their storage as fat.

Three Techniques for Measuring Body Fat

There are several popular methods for measuring body fat. Following are three of the most popular:

1. *Hydrostatic weighing,* in which a person's mass is measured both in and out of a tank of water, is considered to be the gold standard for measuring body fat. This test is based on the assumption that lean tissue is denser than fat—that is, lean tissue will sink and fat tissue will float. This test costs between $100 and $150 and can be performed at your local health club, hospital, university, or wellness center. Some mobile units may even charge as little as $45 for this service.
2. *Skin fold measurement with a caliper* involves measuring subcutaneous (under-the-skin) fat with a caliper at certain points on the body. Since this test has been around for quite some time, you can get it done at YMCAs, health clubs, dietitians' offices, physical therapy centers, and universities.
3. *Anthropometric measurement* is a test you can do at home. This test is based on the assumption that fat is distributed at certain sites on the body such as the neck, wrist, and waistline. Muscle tissue is usually found at sites such as the biceps, forearm, and calf.

The following two anthropometric tests—one for males and one for females—will help you ascertain your percentage of body fat. These formulas are from Philip L. Goglia's book, *Turn Up the Heat: Unlock the Fat-Burning Power of Your Metabolism,* and have a plus or minus error rate of 5 percent. All you need is a cloth tape measure and a calculator.

AT-HOME BODY FAT TEST FOR MALES

Step 1: Taking Measurements

1. Height in inches ____
2. Hips in inches ____
3. Waist in inches ____
4. Weight in pounds ____

Step 2: Determining Your Percentage of Body Fat

1. Multiply your hips (in.) ____ $\times$ 1.4 = ____ minus 2 = ____ (A)
2. Multiply your waist (in.) ____ $\times$ 0.72 = ____ minus 4 = ____ (B)
3. Add A plus B = ____ (C)
4. Multiply your height (in.) ____ $\times$ 0.61 = ____ (D)
5. Subtract D from C, then subtract 10 more: (C – D) – 10 = ____ % fat

Your answer will be your approximate body fat percentage if you are a male.

AT-HOME BODY FAT TEST FOR FEMALES

Step 1: Taking Measurements

1. Height in inches ____
2. Hips in inches ____
3. Waist in inches ____
4. Weight in pounds ____

Step 2: Determining Your Percentage of Body Fat

1. Multiply your hips (in.) ____ $\times$ 1.4 = ____ minus 1 = ____ (A)
2. Multiply your waist (in.) ____ $\times$ 0.72 = ____ minus 2 = ____ (B)
3. Add A plus B = ____ (C)
4. Multiply your height (in.) ____ $\times$ 0.61 = ____ (D)
5. Subtract D from C, then subtract 10 more: (C – D) – 10 = ____ % fat

Your answer will be your approximate body fat percentage if you are a female.

You do not necessarily have to get your body fat tested to know that your body composition is improving. If you have been exercising and eating properly and your clothes begin to feel looser, if you find yourself taking in your belt a notch or two, or if you observe increased strength and muscularity, you will know that you are losing fat and gaining lean muscle.

Calculate Pounds of Body Fat and Lean Muscle

The final step is to take your total weight and calculate how many pounds of fat you carry and how many pounds of lean muscle. Use the following two formulas:

Total weight (lb.) × percent body fat = total pounds of fat

Total weight – total pounds of fat = total pounds of lean muscle

For example, if you are a woman weighing 200 pounds and you find that you have 35 percent body fat, calculate the number of pounds of fat you carry using the following formula:

200 lb. × .35 (% body fat) = 70 pounds of fat

To calculate your pounds of lean muscle, use the following formula:

200 lb. – 70 lb. of fat = 130 pounds of lean muscle

Health Criterion #3: All-over Body Measurements

As you work through the twelve-week Fat-Burning Metabolic Fitness Plan, your all-over body measurements, which I will ask you to take every four weeks, will be another indication that you are losing fat and building lean muscle. You will become leaner and trimmer.

To take accurate all-over body measurements, follow these instructions. I have provided drawings for both men and women to help you to accurately measure each area of your body.

Arm: With your arm to the side of your body, measure the circumference midway between the shoulder and the elbow.

Forearm: With your arm hanging downward and slightly away from your trunk and your palm facing forward, measure at the maximum forearm circumference between the wrist and the elbow.

Chest: For a woman, measure across the widest part of the chest marked by the nipples. (For older women with very large hanging breasts, this might be slightly higher. See illustration for guidance.)

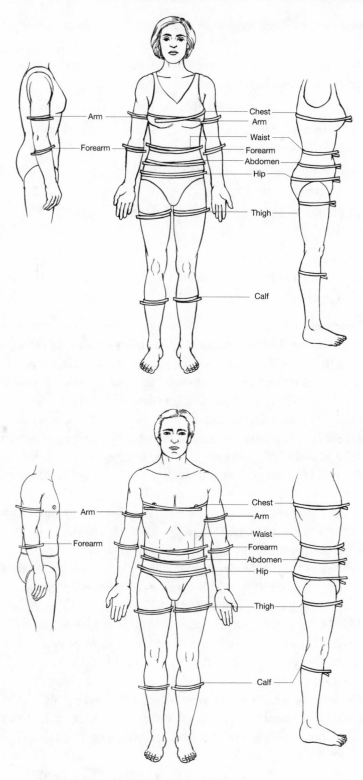

For a man, measure the widest area of the chest across the nipples.

Waist: Measure at the narrowest part of the torso, above the belly button and below the rib cage.

Abdomen: Measure at the level of the belly button.

Hips: Measure at the maximum circumference of the hips or buttocks region, whichever is larger.

Thigh: With your legs slightly apart, measure at the maximum circumference of the thigh.

Calf: Measure at the maximum circumference between the knee and the ankle.

Health Criterion #4: Why Waist Circumference Is So Important

In both men and women, one of the most important and accurate indicators of obesity, the potential for cardiac disease, and other health risks is the circumference of the waist. This is because an increased measurement in the waist always indicates an increase in abdominal fat (and the ratio of body fat–to–lean muscle in general). For a woman, who naturally carries her fat in her hips and thighs, an increased waist measurement indicates a reverse fat pattern.

Since fat is three times the size of lean muscle tissue, it is possible for scale weight and BMI to remain the same with aging yet for the waist to increase as lean muscle is lost and fat storage is increased through inactivity and poor nutritional habits. One doctor I know had a 7-inch increase in his waistline after retirement even though his scale weight did not change.

In the book *It Can Break Your Heart*, Dr. J. Pervis Milnor III and coauthors write that a waistline greater than 35 inches in a woman and 40 inches in a man increases the risk for developing higher cholesterol levels, which lead to coronary disease, and type 2 diabetes. According to the National Heart, Lung and Blood Institute, a man whose waistline is 42 inches or greater is more likely to have erectile dysfunction than his leaner counterparts.

Of course, a waist measurement of 35 inches in women or 40 inches in men is not always an absolute indicator of health risks. You should take into consideration factors such as height, body type, and bone structure. A 35-inch waistline on a woman who is 5 feet 11 inches tall with a large frame would represent less of a health risk than the same waist circumference on a woman who is 5 feet 2 inches tall with a small frame.

Health Criterion #5: Calculate Your Waist-to-Hip Ratio

The value of the waist-to-hip ratio is that it helps to give you a more accurate idea of where you carry your fat. When fat is stored around and above the waist, it results in a higher risk for diabetes, heart disease, and some types of cancers. The person with upper body fat distribution (the apple shape) loses fat more quickly than the person with lower body fat distribution (the pear shape), but a smaller amount of fat stored above the waist is more dangerous than a larger amount of fat stored below the waist.

To get this ratio, measure your waist at its narrowest circumference and your hips at their widest. Then divide your waist measurement by your hip measurement. For example, if you have a waist of 30 inches and a hip measurement of 42 inches, your hip-to-waist ratio is 0.71.

My waist measurement is ____. My hip measurement is ____. My waist-to-hip ratio is ____.

RANGE OF WAIST-TO-HIP RATIOS

	Excellent	Good	Average	High	Extreme
Male	<0.85	0.85–0.9	0.91–0.95	0.96–1.0	>1.0
Female	<0.75	0.75–0.8	0.81–0.85	0.86–0.9	>0.9

Keep in mind that this measurement does not tell you anything about your total body weight or body composition. It just gives you an indication of where your excess fat is located and therefore your health risk relative to fat deposition.

Women must especially watch this ratio during and following menopause when hormonal fluctuations, poor nutrition, and lack of activity can result in abdominal weight gain, leading to a reverse fat pattern. The National Cancer Institute has shown that a woman with a lower than normal waist-to-hip ratio is eight times more likely to get cervical cancer than a woman with a normal ratio.

Used alone, this ratio can be deceiving in some people. As we have seen, once abdominal obesity sets in, especially as a reverse fat pattern, the waist-to-hip ratio can become skewed because at this point both genders are gaining weight above and below the waist. So as the waistline goes up, the hips go up, often in tandem. This is just another reason why no single method of measuring fat storage is infallible. It is important to look at the bigger picture when evaluating your health and fat patterns.

Health Criterion #6: Body Mass Index

The Body Mass Index or BMI is another important tool to help ascertain how overfat you are. Sometimes the BMI can be misleading. For example, a 240-pound bodybuilder who is 5 feet 11 inches would have a BMI of 34, which would appear to put him in the very highest risk category. But if that same person has only 8 percent body fat, this changes the entire story.

However, for most readers of this book, a high BMI will be a red flag predicting many health risks. For example, a recent study published by the American College of Sports Medicine has shown a direct correlation between a high BMI and increased levels of C-reactive protein. High CRP is an accurate indicator of inflammation in the body, which increases the risk of a first cardiac event (heart attack), even after adjustments have been made for risk factors such as age, smoking, and body weight. Exercise and increased levels of physical activity, which result in weight loss and lowered BMI, have been shown to reduce a person's level of CRP. So while the BMI is not an infallible standard by which to measure how fat you are, taken together with other factors it is a useful tool for helping to create an accurate health profile and can serve as an early warning system for heart disease.

BMI is defined as your weight in kilograms divided by your height in meters squared. To save you the trouble of converting pounds to kilograms and inches to meters, I have done the math for you. Simply look up your BMI in the chart provided. Your height can be found in the left-hand column and your weight (in pounds) runs along the top of the chart. Your BMI is where both points intersect. Because people between 5 feet and 5 feet 2 inches tall generally have a lighter frame, we have included a different chart for them.

Interpret Your BMI

- *If your BMI is below 20.* Unless you are an athlete with a very high ratio of lean muscle–to–body fat, a BMI this low might mean that you are too thin and are possibly compromising your immune system.
- *If your BMI is between 20 and 22.* This range is associated with living the longest and having the lowest incidence of serious illness.
- *If your BMI is between 23 and 25.* These numbers are still within the acceptable range and are associated with good health.
- *If your BMI is between 26 and 30.* Now you are entering the zone where there are serious health risks. A BMI this high puts you at risk

BODY MASS INDEX

	100	110	120	130	140	150	160	170	180	190	200	210	220	230	240	250	260	270	280
5'0"	20	22	24	26	27	29	31	33	35	37	39	41	43	45	47	49	51	53	55
5'1"	19	21	23	25	27	28	30	32	34	37	39	41	43	45	47	49	51	53	55
5'2"	19	20	22	24	26	28	29	31	33	35	36	37	39	41	43	44	46	48	50

	120	130	140	150	160	170	180	190	200	210	220	230	240	250	260	270	280	290	300
5'3"	21	23	25	27	28	30	32	34	36	37	39	41	43	44	46	48	50	51	53
5'4"	21	22	24	26	28	29	31	33	34	36	38	40	41	43	45	46	48	50	52
5'5"	20	22	23	25	27	28	30	32	33	35	37	38	40	42	43	45	47	48	50
5'6"	19	21	23	24	26	27	29	31	32	34	36	37	39	40	42	44	45	47	49
5'7"	19	20	22	24	25	27	28	30	31	33	35	36	38	39	41	42	44	46	47
5'8"	18	20	21	23	24	26	27	29	30	32	34	35	37	38	40	41	43	44	46
5'9"	18	19	21	22	24	25	27	28	30	31	33	34	36	37	38	40	41	43	44
5'10"	17	19	20	22	23	24	26	27	29	30	32	33	35	36	37	39	40	42	43
5'11"	17	18	20	21	22	24	25	27	28	29	31	32	34	35	36	38	39	41	42
6'0"	16	18	19	20	22	23	24	26	27	29	30	31	33	34	35	37	38	39	41
6'1"	16	17	19	20	21	22	24	25	26	28	29	30	32	33	34	36	37	38	40
6'2"	15	17	18	19	21	22	23	24	26	27	28	30	31	32	33	35	36	37	39
6'3"	15	16	18	19	20	21	23	24	25	26	28	29	30	31	33	34	35	36	38
6'4"	15	16	17	18	20	21	22	23	24	26	27	28	29	30	32	33	34	35	37
6'5"	14	15	17	18	19	20	21	23	24	25	26	27	29	30	31	32	33	34	36
6'6"	14	15	16	17	19	20	21	22	23	24	25	27	28	29	30	31	32	34	35

for developing heart disease, stroke, type 2 diabetes, and some kinds of cancers. You should definitely lower your weight through diet and exercise.

- *If your BMI is over 30.* This is the worst-case scenario where you are definitely putting yourself at risk for all of the diseases mentioned above. It is imperative that you begin to lose weight and exercise.

According to a study done in the *New England Journal of Medicine,* having a BMI over 25 may cause your life span to decrease significantly. If your BMI is higher than 30, your life span may decrease even more sharply. Studies show that 59 percent of American men have a BMI over 25 and almost as many women. For those who have a BMI over 35, health care costs are likely to be more than twice those of individuals with a BMI between 20 and 25. Treatment of diabetes, hypertension, and cardiovascular disease count for much of this spending.

Compare Your BMI and Waist Measurement

As we have seen, BMI can be skewed by factors such as frame size and the percentage of lean muscle that you carry on your frame. One tool that I have found useful in deciding whether your BMI is in the healthy range is the comparison between BMI and waist measurement. Here is a chart that compares ranges of BMI with waist measurements in men and women.

RELATIONSHIP BETWEEN BMI AND WAIST MEASUREMENTS

Health Category	BMI	Men's Waist (in.)	Women's Waist (in.)
Normal	18.5–24.9	34.3–38.5	31.1–36.1
Overweight	25–29.9	38.6–42.8	36.2–40.4
Obese I	30–34.9	42.9–48.7	40.5–45.2
Obese II	≥35	≥48.8	≥45.3

If both your BMI and your waistline fall into the same category, you can be fairly certain of the health classification.

Bo Walker: The Inches Melted Off and the Numbers Went Down

Let's take a look at a client of mine who completed the Fat-Burning Metabolic Fitness Plan as part of a makeover I did for *Let's Live* magazine: a forty-year-old radio personality named Bo Walker. When Bo first came into my program, he carried 250 pounds on his 5-foot 10-inch frame, had a body fat percentage of 34.5, a BMI of 35.85, a waist measurement of 48, and a waist-to-hip ratio of 1.0. As you can see, all of these figures put him into the very highest risk category.

Bo was concerned about his health because he and his wife had a young child. "I knew I was headed in the wrong direction. My father had died at a very early age, fifty-nine years old, from a heart attack and complications with diabetes. I knew that if I continued on this path and stayed in the 250 weight range—or worse—I was probably headed for the same fate. I wanted my kid to know who I am and I wanted to live long enough to enjoy my life with my wife." Bo was also facing the stress of having just lost his job.

Over the course of twelve weeks, Bo saw dramatic changes in his overall body measurements. I have included some of his statistics to demonstrate his total transformation.

BO WALKER'S MEASUREMENTS

	Date					
	5/1/2003	5/17/2003	5/31/2003	6/26/2003	7/12/2003	8/1/2003
% Body Fat	34.50	27.80	24.80	23.20	23.20	20.80
BMI	35.85	34.7	33.91	33.41	33.41	32.4
Weight	250	242	236.5	233	233	226
Girths: Left/Right						
Bicep–Left	15	14	13.75	14	13.75	13.5
Bicep–Right	14	14	13.75	13.75	13.75	13.75
Forearm–Left		11.75	11.75	12	12	11.75
Forearm–Right		12	12	12	12	12
Thigh–Left	27	27	25	25.5	25.5	23.5
Thigh–Right	27	26	25	25.25	25	23.75
Calf–Left		16	15.5	15.25	15.25	15
Calf–Right		16.5	16.5	16.25	16.25	16
Hips	46.5	47.5	45.75	45	44.75	42.75
Waist	48	47.5	46.5	45.75	45	43.75
Shoulders		54	52.75	52.5	53	52
Chest	49	49	47.75	46.5	46.5	45.25

As you can see, Bo lost 24 pounds and his body fat dropped 13.7 points, from 34.5 percent to 20.8 percent. If we plug this into the formula I gave you, he started out carrying 86.5 pounds of fat and 163.5 pounds of lean muscle. At the end of 12 weeks, he was carrying only 47 pounds of fat and 179 pounds of lean muscle—a dramatic change. If you interpret these figures from a slightly different perspective, in terms of conversion from fat to muscle, Bo lost 39.5 pounds of fat and gained 15.5 pounds of lean muscle. Quite impressive!

All of Bo's other measurements decreased as well. His BMI dropped from 35.85 to 32.4 and his waistline shrunk from 48 to 43.75, a loss of 4.25 inches. His hip measurement dropped from 46.5 to 42.75, a loss of 3.75 inches, resulting in a waist-to-hip ratio of 1.0, which is identical to his former ratio. This is a perfect example of the shortcomings of looking only at this measurement, as discussed earlier in this chapter. As I explained, when taken alone, the waist-to-hip ratio is not a reliable indicator of health risk. When a man has developed a reverse fat pattern, as Bo did, at first the waist and hips will shrink in tandem with one another as the body is normalizing.

In extreme cases of the reverse fat pattern, such as Douglas Daniels, the waist-to-hip ratio will actually increase before it goes down. The reason is that the hips are not a normal place for a man to store fat. The rule is that the last fat gained is the first to be lost.

Bo still has a distance to go, but he looks and feels better than he has in years, which is a strong motivator for him to continue with the plan. Your body could also look great after only four weeks on the Fat-Burning Metabolic Fitness Plan.

5

Learn How to Interpret Your Blood Work

Before you begin the Fat-Burning Metabolic Fitness Plan, ask your doctor to draw your blood and do a full metabolic profile. If you decide to take advantage of your higher metabolic rate and fat-burning ability and continue beyond the basic four-week plan into Modules 2 and 3, you might wish to repeat this test at the twelve-week mark so that you can see how dramatically the nutritional and exercise programs have improved your cholesterol, triglycerides, and glucose levels. You can plug the numbers from your lab work into the following profile:

Metabolic Lab Analysis Questionnaire

HDL _____
LDL _____
Triglycerides _____
Total Cholesterol _____
Ratio between Your Total Cholesterol and Your HDL _____

Lipoprotein (a) _____
High-Sensitivity C-reactive Protein _____
Glucose _____

Learn How to Interpret Your Full Lipid Profile

While people are aware that they should get their cholesterol checked, most do not know much about how to interpret the results. Before you fill out this profile, there are certain terms related to your blood chemistry that you should understand. When your doctor does a full lipid profile, he or she is evaluating five basic numbers.

1. *High-density lipoprotein (HDL)* is the type of cholesterol that we think of as good or protective. If small amounts of plaque (LDL or bad cholesterol) have been laid down in your blood vessels and you have enough HDL, you will be able to dissolve this plaque and use it as an energy source.
   - Good HDL is 40 mg/dl and above for man.
   - Good HDL is 50 mg/dl and above for a woman.
2. *Low-density lipoprotein (LDL)* is the bad type of cholesterol that collects in your blood vessels as plaque and clogs them if you have too much floating around in your bloodstream or if you don't have sufficient HDL to dissolve it. According to the new cholesterol standards for both genders recently published by the *Journal of the American Medical Association*:
   - An LDL of less than 100 mg/dl is optimal.
   - 100–129 mg/dl is near or above optimal.
   - 130–159 mg/dl is borderline high.
   - 160–189 mg/dl is high.
   - 190 mg/dl and up is very high.
3. *Triglycerides* are the fats that appear in the blood immediately after a meal or snack. Normally, they are stripped of their fatty acids when they pass through various types of tissue, especially adipose (beneath the skin) fat and skeletal muscle. When this happens, they are converted into stored energy that is gradually released and metabolized between meals according to the metabolic needs of your body. Almost everyone loves sugars and other kinds of carbohydrates. Unfortunately, if you are insulin sensitive and eat more carbohydrates than you require daily, your triglyceride level will elevate. When this happens, your disease risk for hypoglycemia and type 2 diabetes can increase and you will become more susceptible to coronary disease.
   - A normal triglyceride level is 150 or below.
   - 150–199 is borderline high.
   - 200–499 is high.
   - 500 or over is very high.
4. Your *total cholesterol* is found by adding your HDL plus your LDL plus your triglycerides divided by 5. Ideally, your total cholesterol should be 100 plus your age.

- A total cholesterol less than 200 mg/dl is desirable.
- 200–239 mg/dl is borderline high.
- 240 mg/dl or greater is considered high.

5. Another important number in your full lipid profile is the *ratio between your total cholesterol and your HDL.*
   - The average male has a 3.5:1 ratio.
   - The average female has a 4.5:1 ratio.
   - The average athlete has a 2.1:1 to 2.8:1 ratio.

Newer Blood Markers for Health Risks

One of the newer markers for health risks is a test for lipoprotein (a). Lp(a) is a substance that is structurally very similar to LDL. Although your Lp(a) values are influenced by genetics, levels are generally higher in African Americans and in women. The elderly seem to have higher levels as well. A recent study of nearly 6,000 individuals conducted at Johns Hopkins University Hospital showed that men over age sixty-five with the highest levels of Lp(a) had three times the risk of stroke and death from cardiovascular disease than individuals with lower levels.

Elevated levels of Lp(a) may increase vascular disease risk by inhibiting the body's ability to dissolve clots, by playing a role in "foam cell" formation (an early step in the atherosclerosis process), and by increasing oxidative stress. Oxidative stress is often referred to as the body's rust and can be seen in the little brown age marks that you have on the back of your hands. Since it is a member of the cholesterol family, Lp(a) can form fatty plaques that can block arteries. Although most studies have shown that an elevated Lp(a) alone is a risk factor for cardiovascular disease, your risk will be particularly increased when you also have elevated total cholesterol or LDL levels.

Another of the newer markers for risk factors is *high-sensitivity C-reactive protein.* Hs-CRP is a very accurate indicator for small levels of inflammation in the body. Low levels of inflammation often accompany atherosclerosis and are usually present to a greater degree in individuals likely to develop future heart attacks and strokes. In studies of healthy men and women, as well as those who already have heart disease, hs-CRP has been shown to be at least as strong, if not stronger, than cholesterol measurements in predicting future heart attack and stroke. When you combine measurements of cholesterol with your hs-CRP score and your other risk factors, the ability to predict your risk of future heart attack increases markedly. Both of these tests are fairly inexpensive and should be covered by most health plans.

If you have your blood work redone at the end of twelve weeks, do not be surprised if your Lp(a) and hs-CRP values do not change much. They are really only considered to be markers for possible risk factors and change very slowly over time.

Metabolic Syndrome X

Now that you have done the self-evaluation work in this chapter and chapter 4, you have all of the information you need to see if you suffer from the cluster of symptoms that doctors have labeled as Metabolic Syndrome X. One of the most dangerous problems with fat in the abdominal area, especially in men and women over age forty, is that it lays the groundwork for this syndrome. The main characteristic of Metabolic Syndrome X is an increasing resistance to insulin, eventually leading to type 2 diabetes and in some cases type 1 diabetes. According to the American Diabetes Association, type 2 diabetes and the distribution of fat in the abdominal area are directly related to cardiovascular disease and stroke.

There are five main measurements that are listed as risk factors for Metabolic Syndrome X. To be at risk, you have to have three out of five of the symptoms listed below. If you do not know your blood pressure, you can either get it tested at your doctor's office or in most drugstores where they offer self-tests.

Metabolic Syndrome X Questionnaire

	Yes	No
1. Do you have a waist circumference greater than 40 inches if you are a man or greater than 35 inches if you are a woman?	☐	☐
2. Do you have hypertension that is being medically treated or blood pressure greater than 135 over 85 mm/Hg?	☐	☐
3. Are your triglycerides greater than 150 mg/dl?	☐	☐
4. Do you have a low HDL value—that is, less than 40 mg/dl if you are a man or less than 50 mg/dl if you are a woman?	☐	☐
5. Do you have a fasting glucose greater than 110 mg/dl?	☐	☐

Carrie: Amazing Changes in Her Lipid Profile

Carrie was forty-eight years old when she started my plan because she wanted to lose about 20 pounds. Although she had once been very active, jogging and going to weekly yoga and dance classes, she had become fairly sedentary in the last seven years. Carrie was especially concerned about the amount of fat she had gained in her abdominal area because she had read about the health risks associated with abdominal fat. She wanted to halt the trend of her fat gain before it became a serious problem.

Carrie was in for some unpleasant surprises. While no one would have considered a 5-foot 8-inch-tall woman to be obese at 158 pounds, Carrie discovered that she had a body fat percentage of 34.5, which put her into a high-risk classification. She thought she knew a lot about good nutrition, but when we evaluated what she was eating, we saw that she was trying to eat mostly vegetarian meals and not doing a very good job of balancing out the three food groups. Her diet consisted mainly of salads mixed with small amounts of tuna, cheese, breads, too many desserts, and pasta, with an occasional chicken breast or omelet thrown in for good measure. When I explained to her why she should be eating 30 percent acceptable fats, 40 percent low-glycemic carbohydrates, and 30 percent lean protein, it was a revelation. She had been suffering from frequent colds and flu and didn't realize how she was compromising her immune system by eating only small amounts of protein.

Since Carrie had stopped jogging to save her joints and had moved away from the city where her dance classes were located, she had stopped exercising except for walking about four times per week. She had read enough to know that if she continued on her present path, her health would deteriorate when she entered menopause, so she was determined to change her lifestyle, eating habits, and approach to exercise.

Carrie's lipid profile was actually pretty good. Her total cholesterol was 193, her LDL was 102, her HDL was 70, her triglycerides were 96, and her glucose was 99. But everything is relative. I have noticed several things over the last two decades. People who are approaching middle life and rapidly gaining fat in the abdominal area, especially women, are not going to have a good lipid profile for long. Carrie's high body fat and her low metabolism from poor nutrition and little exercise were about to tip the scales toward higher cholesterol and triglycerides. With the gain in fat around her waist, she was definitely headed for a reverse fat pattern. I have also noticed that people like Carrie who have acceptable cholesterol and triglycerides even though they carry a large amount of body fat should really have superior lipid values, not just good or borderline values. In Carrie's case, we saw how true this was because her values dropped significantly with weight loss.

As soon as Carrie began to follow a nutritionally balanced, low-glycemic food plan and my program of resistive exercise and interval training, she began to lose fat dramatically. After four weeks on my Fat-Burning Metabolic Fitness Plan, her scale weight was 149 pounds, her body fat was 27.8, her total cholesterol had dropped to 174, her LDL was 114, her HDL was 48, her triglycerides were 60, and her glucose was 103. After twelve weeks on my program, she saw even more dramatic changes. Her weight dropped to 136 pounds and her body fat to 20.5 percent. This represents a loss of 22 scale pounds but actually works out to a loss of 26.7 pounds of fat and a gain of 5.8 pounds of lean muscle. So in just twelve weeks Carrie exceeded her original goal.

When she had her blood work redone, she was astonished to see that her total cholesterol had dropped further to 137, her LDL to 61, her HDL had risen to 66, her triglycerides had dropped to 52, and her glucose to 84. Few people can brag of having an LDL lower than their HDL. Her numbers were as good as those of any Olympic athlete.

With a body fat percentage of 20.5, Carrie had dropped from a size 12 dress to a size 6. She told me, "I had no idea that eating and exercising right would make such a dramatic difference." Whenever someone in her family comes back from their yearly physical with high cholesterol and triglycerides, she tells them about my program. Recently she told me, "My brother in Pennsylvania called and said that he had been to his doctor. He had gained 30 pounds, his triglycerides were 300, and his cholesterol was 323. I read him the riot act! Then I went right down the list with him, coaching him with everything you had taught me and promising to send him a copy of your books *Lose Your Love Handles* and *Maximum Energy for Life*. Yesterday he called me back and told me that he had lost 16 pounds, his triglycerides had dropped to 156, and his cholesterol was now 232, just from following your program. Thank you, Mackie."

Carrie was smart enough to recognize that her fat was rapidly migrating from below the belt up to her midsection. Even though her body fat was getting very high, she caught herself before she developed serious health problems. She is now on my maintenance plan and feels great. A few months ago she told me that she had just celebrated her fiftieth birthday. "I may have hit the big five-oh, but I feel better now than I ever have in my life. What a great way to make my debut into middle age."

6

Your Thyroid and Human Growth Hormone

Even though 10 million Americans have been diagnosed with thyroid problems, millions more live with lethargy, muscle weakness, depression, menstrual irregularities, low sex drive, and weight gain due to an undiagnosed thyroid condition. Doctors used to estimate that as many as 13 million people had some form of hypo- or hyperthyroidism and didn't know it. However, at an international Consensus Development Conference held by the College of Integrative Medicine in 2003, the number of undiagnosed cases was reported to be closer to 50 million if looking at the whole clinical picture, which includes not just the standard lab tests but the physical exam, the patient's symptoms, and his or her basal body temperature. This was in alignment with the position taken by the late Dr. Broda Barnes, a well-known pioneer in the field of thyroid disease and author of *Hypothyroidism, the Unsuspected Illness.* Barnes estimated that at one time or another approximately 40 percent of the population will suffer from clinical hypothyroidism.

What Does the Thyroid Gland Do?

The thyroid is the master gland at regulating metabolism. It is a small butterfly-shaped gland wrapped around the windpipe behind and below the Adam's apple area. The thyroid produces two key hormones, triiodothyronine (T3) and thryroxine (T4), which act like engines, getting oxygen into every cell in your body so that your cells get the energy they need to function.

When the thyroid is functioning properly, 80 percent of the hormones it releases will be T4 and 20 percent T3, which is considered to be the more biologically active of the two. The liver, the kidney, and the cells further break down T4 into T3.

Hypothyroidism means that the thyroid is underactive, and hyperthyroidism means that it is overactive. An enlarged thyroid gland is often called a goiter. Sometimes an inflammation of the thyroid gland (Hashimoto's disease) will cause significant enlargement of the gland.

Since hyperthyroidism is not as prevalent and its symptoms are fairly easy to spot—bulging eyes, racing heart, profuse sweating, nervousness, and jittery feelings most of the time—I will focus on helping you to recognize if you might be suffering from the great metabolic shutdown associated with hypothyroidism.

What's Wrong with the Lab Tests?

If you go to your doctor to have your thyroid tested, he or she will draw your blood and send it to the lab to obtain a thyroid panel. While the advances made in diagnosing diseases in the laboratory have been remarkable over the last decade, as can be seen in the tests for illnesses such as rheumatoid arthritis and breast cancer, lab tests for hypothyroid problems are still largely inaccurate, according to Dr. Charles Mary III of the Mary Clinic in Louisiana. Dr. Mary's position was backed up by the majority of doctors attending the recent Consensus Development Conference.

One of the breakthroughs in the last several decades has been the Thyroid Stimulating Hormone (TSH) test. When doctors first discovered how to measure this hormone, they decided that TSH was the gold standard of diagnosing thyroid dysfunction. TSH is a hormone produced by the pituitary gland in response to fluctuations of thyroid hormone. If the brain sees low levels of thyroid hormones in the body, or if a person's metabolism is poor, the brain will begin to pump out higher levels of TSH. So, according to this lab test, elevated TSH would be indicative of hypothyroid function.

According to Mario McNally, MD, an endocrinologist, and James Carter, MD, DrPH, the emeritus head of the Nutrition Section at Tulane University School of Public Health and Tropical Medicine, the problem is that a person can be very ill with hypothyroidism yet still have a normal TSH test—that is, it is still possible for someone to have hypothyroidism when his or her levels of TSH are low. When the lab work shows that TSH is in the low or normal range in these cases, the problem is that the body is not adequately converting the hormone T4 to T3. Remember, T3 is a crucial hormone in getting oxygen into the cells and in enabling efficient metabolic function.

Factors that inhibit the body's conversion of T4 to T3 are low levels of iodine, selenium, zinc, copper, vitamin B12, vitamin B6, vitamin A, and vitamin E; high levels of fluoride; high or low levels of serum ferritin; and a diet that is too low in calories. Other factors that interfere with the conversion of T4 to T3 are beta-blockers, birth-control pills, high levels of estrogen, lithium, lead, mercury, stress, cigarette smoking, pesticides, aging, diabetes, surgery, adrenal insufficiency, and human growth hormone deficiency.

According to Dr. Mary, one of the main hormones that impairs the efficiency of the conversion of T4 to T3 is estrogen. He suggests that the widespread use of birth-control pills and hormone replacement therapy (HRT) drugs such as Premarin may be contributing to our epidemic of obesity by making it harder for the body to convert T4 to T3. As evidence, he points out that all farmers know that you can easily fatten up cows, pigs, chickens, and other animals by giving them estrogen. Dr. Mary has found that 90 percent of the patients he diagnoses with hypothyroidism are women.

How Do I Know If I Have Hypothyroidism?

According to the *Consensus Report of the International College of Integrative Medicine,* there are two main approaches to accurately diagnosing a patient with hypothyroidism. The first approach is the comprehensive thyroid panel, which includes testing for ultrasensitive TSH (levels lower than 3.04, which is the usual accepted low end of normal in the regular TSH test), and levels of T4, free T4, T3, free T3, and reverse T3. This test has the advantage of allowing your doctor to look at the interrelationships between the different levels of hormones. It's not just one factor that determines healthy thyroid function but the synergistic relationship between several hormones.

According the to *Consensus Report,* the second and most effective approach to making an accurate diagnosis of thyroid problems is to consider the lab work as a backup but to base the main part of the diagnosis on taking a patient's history, doing a thorough physical exam, recording basal axillary temperatures, and checking the Achilles reflex. All of these taken together constitute a more complete (holistic) approach to the diagnosis and treatment of hypothyroidism.

When we are evaluating a new client who seems highly symptomatic, my doctors always check for thyroid problems because trying to boost a person's metabolism when he or she is suffering from severe thyroid problems is like asking someone to run a race with a bowling ball tied to his or her foot. Hypothyroidism is too complex for you to self-diagnose from a chapter in a book. But the following hypothyroid questionnaire created by Dr. Mary can guide you as to whether you should consult with an endocrinologist. You may have hypothyroidism if you check off about eight of these symptoms. However, as Dr. Mary points out, a person might only present with one symptom such as depression or low body temperature upon awakening in the morning.

SIGNS AND SYMPTOMS OF HYPOTHYROIDISM

_____ Loss of Appetite

_____ Weakness

_____ Dry Skin

_____ Edema (Swelling) of Eyelids

_____ Cold Skin

_____ Edema of Face

_____ Heart Enlargement

_____ Impaired Memory

_____ Gain in Weight

_____ Pallor of Lips

_____ Deafness

_____ Nervousness

_____ Labored or Difficult Breathing

_____ Palpitations

_____ Pain Over Heart

_____ Painful Menstruation

_____ Emotional Instability

_____ Fineness of Hair

_____ Depression

_____ Muscle Pain

_____ Heat Intolerance

_____ Slowing of Mental Activity

_____ Burning or Tingling Sensation

_____ Cyanosis (Bluish Discoloration of Skin)

_____ Lethargy

_____ Coarse Skin

_____ Slow Speech

_____ Sensation of Cold

_____ Thick Tongue

_____ Coarseness of Hair

_____ Pallor of Skin

_____ Constipation

_____ Loss of Hair

_____ Swelling of Feet

_____ Excessive Menstruation

_____ Hoarseness

_____ Decreased Sweating

_____ Poor Heart Sounds

_____ Changes in Back of Eye

_____ Loss of Weight

_____ Choking Sensation

_____ Brittle Nails

_____ Muscle Weaknes

_____ Joint Pain

_____ Slow Movements

_____ Difficulty in Swallowing

_____ Poor Vision

_____ **Total Answers**

What Is the Most Effective Treatment for Hypothyroidism?

It used to be that patients with hypothyroidism were given desiccated (dehydrated) pig's liver, but this medication was replaced by newer synthetic products. One of the most widely used is a drug called Synthroid. Although patients on Synthroid often improve with a lowering of their TSH, they often reach a plateau where they still have many of the signs and symptoms of hypothyroidism. Dr. Mary explains that synthetic thyroid medications supply the body with T4 only. "If you can't convert T4 to T3, you are going to have inadequate levels of T3 in the body, even though you have normal levels of T4. The way to overcome this is to just give them the combination therapy, with both T4 and T3." For this reason, Dr. Mary and many of the endocrinologists with whom I consult have been going back to an older and highly respected thyroid medication called Armour Thyroid. This medication is made from desiccated pig's liver and contains both T3 and T4. According to the *Consensus Report,* doctors agreed that "patients will continue to improve when switched to desiccated thyroid."

Three Steps to Help Prevent or Minimize Hypothyroidism

Step 1: Exercise on a Regular Basis

In *Dr. Murray's Total Body Tune-up,* he writes, "When we're not exercising, it's the body's cue to more or less hibernate. The thyroid gland is the major organ of metabolism and if you're not exercising your metabolism slows and, as a result, the thyroid gland starts functioning at a lower level as well."

While most of the endocrinologists with whom I consulted for this book told me that there was no natural cure for hypothyroidism, they were all in agreement that a good program of exercise could help prevent thyroid problems and would certainly help to strengthen the effects of any thyroid medication. The reasons are twofold.

First, hypothyroidism develops when several of the body's hormones are out of balance, especially estrogen, which inhibits the ability to convert T4 to T3. I have seen literally hundreds of men and women with thyroid problems improve dramatically when they began following my Fat-Burning Metabolic Fitness Plan because research shows that appropriate exercise helps to balance out the body hormonally. Douglas Daniels is an excellent example. He came into the program with undiagnosed hypothyroidism but began to experience significant results and a much better quality of life after two weeks of exercise, at which point he started taking thyroid medication.

Second, we are looking at a "What came first, the chicken or the egg?" situation when we look at the metabolic condition of someone with hypothyroidism. A person who has developed an inefficient metabolism because he never exercises is setting himself up for hormonal imbalances. One of the main characteristics of someone with a sluggish metabolism is a lower than normal body temperature. According to the *Consensus Report,* enzymes are very temperature sensitive, as are other bodily functions. If a person is not metabolically fit—running the engine on cool, if you will—he or she will not have a proper hormonal balance. The less efficient thyroid function becomes, the less efficient metabolism becomes, creating a downward spiral.

However, as Dr. Mary points out, once you develop hypothyroidism, it is very simple and inexpensive to take Armour Thyroid. Problems such as obesity, joint pain, depression, and chronic exhaustion make exercising harder. Finding relief from these problems can help a person to find the energy to stay on a good exercise program.

Step 2: Eat Nutritionally

Dr. Mary states that the number one reason that people develop hypothyroidism is because something is blocking the natural function of the thyroid. "If we cleared our systems of all of the garbage, if we had the ability to eat pure organic meat, pure unadulterated vegetables, to maintain an ideal body weight, to drink pure water, and breathe pure air—then we could eliminate some of the issues that are blocking proper thyroid function." While Dr. Mary feels that eating organic vegetables and hormone-free meat can sometimes seem like a monumental task, I have seen over and over again how easy it is to maintain a healthy eating plan once you have made it a part of your daily regimen. Eating nutritionally takes some thought and planning in the beginning, but it soon becomes habit. Fortunately, we live in an enlightened time when supermarkets and food chains are offering a wide selection of healthier and more natural food choices.

Step 3: Get Proper Supplementation

Ideally we should be able to get all of the vitamins and minerals from the foods we eat, but there are two factors working against that. The first is that we cook most of our foods, which destroys essential nutrients. The second and most important is that we are growing our food in soil that is often exhausted of certain vital minerals. According to Dr. Mary, "U.S. Geological Survey maps from 50 years ago will tell us that there's no more magnesium in the soil now compared to what it was. There are entire communities filled with people that have heart problems because their soil has selenium deficiencies. Eighty percent of a community with heart disease? That's bizarre. So, nutritional depletions in our foodstuffs are rampant and I think that's why people need to supplement. And supplementation is not as easy as just popping into your local pharmacy and picking up Centrum."

Well-known naturopath Dr. Michael Murray suggests a basic supplementation program for thyroid health. He writes: "I am a firm believer in building a strong foundation. In that goal, there are three key dietary supplements that I recommend to provide a strong foundation for a proper nutritional supplement plan:

- A high-potency multiple vitamin and mineral formula (MultiStart).
- A 'greens' drink product (Enriching Greens).
- A pharmaceutical grade fish oil supplement (RxOmega-3 Factors)."

Dr. Murray recommends his specially designed vitamin/mineral supplement MultiStart because it contains optimal levels of zinc, copper, manganese, and the vitamins A, B2, B3, B6, C, and E (MultiStart is available in most health food stores or on the Internet). Deficiencies of any of these substances "could cause or contribute to hypothyroidism." I have found this to be a wonderful product, but any high-quality multivitamin/mineral that you can buy in a health food store will include these nutrients. Just remember to read labels carefully before you buy vitamins.

Again, these three steps will help prevent thyroid problems and will greatly help in minimizing the symptoms of mild cases of hypothyroidism. However, low thyroid function is a serious problem. If you suspect that you are hypothyroid, make an appointment with an endocrinologist who will do more than just a basic lab test. A natural thyroid medication may be needed to help balance out your hormones and increase your metabolic efficiency.

The Lifestyle Deficits of Borderline Hypothyroidism

Allie, a twenty-four-year-old actress, came into my program because she was overweight and was suffering from some quality-of-life issues. Her doctor had told her that she was borderline hypothyroid but had left her untreated. I could see that she had all of the classic symptoms of hypothyroidism: she was overweight, felt tired all the time, and had trouble concentrating and sleeping at night. When we ran a metabolic study on her, which has an error factor built into it of plus or minus 10 percent, we found out that she scored 20 percent below the lowest end of normal. Even allowing for the range of error, that's at least 10 percent too low.

When I sent Allie to Dr. Mary for an evaluation, he felt that she should start on Armour Thyroid. By then Allie had been in the Fat-Burning Metabolic Fitness Plan for two weeks and was already starting to feel significantly better. Now she's been on her thyroid medication for several months and she says, "It has made me feel like a different person."

Allie is a classic example of someone who is hypothyroid but was considered normal and left untreated. Because I encounter clients like Allie quite frequently, I have begun to agree with the doctors who say that low thyroid is an undiagnosed epidemic.

Is Human Growth Hormone Replacement the Answer?

Human growth hormone (HGH) helps to regulate bone and organ growth in your youth. In adulthood, it is responsible for many other metabolic processes including protein synthesis, which means that there is a direct correlation between the level of HGH and the percentage of lean muscle. Many of the obese clients that I see in my program have significantly lower than normal levels of HGH. However, it is normal for this hormone to naturally decrease with age, so no one is going to have the same amount of HGH in middle or old age as he or she had in youth.

Is there anything that can be done about low HGH levels in middle age? A few years ago there was a lot of excitement about HGH injections. Headlines called injectable HGH the fountain of youth. However, interest has begun to wane as people have found out that it is not the simple panacea that it was promised to be.

In fact, every doctor who I asked about HGH injections felt that they are not the answer for several reasons. One is that this therapy is prohibitively expensive, costing $800 to $1,250 per month, and it may not be covered by health insurance. Also, it takes up to six months for these injections to begin to take effect. And, of course, there is the unpleasant prospect of giving yourself a daily injection.

Dr. Michael Murray warns about some of the negative side effects of injectable HGH:

> My take on it is, like most hormones, it's a double-edged sword and needs to be used very carefully if it is being used. I don't know how wise it is to use it. I think there's been a lot of publicity about

its positive benefits. Not enough press has been given to the potential harmful benefits of excess hormone, such as inducing diabetes and actually promoting the growth of cancer and possibly worsening osteoarthritis. Those are some of the risks of excess growth hormone. I'm not too optimistic that HGH injections will be shown to be all that beneficial in the long term. Again, I think that taking into consideration diet and lifestyle and trying to maintain natural levels of HGH for as long as possible is the best way to go. I think there's a reason why the body starts secreting less growth hormone. I think it's a natural process, and any time we go against that process, whether it's growth hormone or whether it's estrogen, we run the risk of doing more harm than good.

As the *Consensus Report* of the International College of Integrative Medicine states, "You can't just focus on one hormone, and the patient has to be treated as a whole person. You have to look at the other aspects of the endocrine system. For example, people with thyroid disorders will not achieve optimal health until the thyroid disorder is corrected first. They may also need testosterone, progesterone, estrogen, etc. So you should check all of the hormone levels when approaching the patient."

Are Secretagogues Safe?

In recent years secretagogues, which act like HGH, have become popular. Like HGH injections, these products come with the promise that they will lower your lipids, increase your muscle mass and strength, and increase your bone mass. However, at a recent meeting of the Consensus Development Conference on Injectable Growth Hormone vs. Growth Hormone Secretagogues hosted by the Great Lakes College of Clinical Medicine, several physicians pointed out that they felt the jury was still out on their effectiveness. These products have been around for only three to five years, and there hasn't been enough time or funding to research their effectiveness.

However, these physicians felt that one advantage that secretagogue supplements may have over injectable HGH is that the hormone isn't injected directly into the bloodstream. It is theorized that secretagogues stimulate the pituitary gland to secrete more HGH, creating more of a balance in the body and making it less likely that a person will end up with too much.

Since I have used a secretagogue with the goal of increasing my own levels of HGH, I tend to disagree that they should be dismissed out of hand. But I do agree that you should be very careful about what kind of secretagogue you take and how often you take it. I only take this supplement daily for a month or two a year because I want to avoid any possible negative side effects. Also, according to Dr. Carter, secretagogues might cause hypertension in certain people, so if you choose to take them, your doctor should monitor your blood pressure for the duration. Secretagogue supplements can be found in any good health food store. Ask your doctor to recommend a brand for you.

How Do I Know If My HGH Levels Are Low?

When I consulted with endocrinologist Dr. Mario McNally about what criteria he used to diagnose low levels of HGH, he gave me five different areas that signaled a deficiency. If you score low in several of these areas, it is likely that you may have low HGH and should consult with your doctor:

1. Body composition—the amount of lean muscle mass compared to fat mass
2. Bone mineral density
3. Exercise capacity
4. Lipid profile
5. Quality-of-life factors

According to Dr. McNally, "The more issues you have in each of these areas, the more likely you are to have an HGH deficiency." Below is Dr. McNally's quality-of-life questionnaire. When I asked him how to score this test, he said that the patient who didn't feel well and who answered yes to the majority of these questions should consider getting a full physical workup by his or her doctor. If the physical and the lab tests show nothing wrong yet the patient still feels badly, has a low sex drive, and has low strength—what doctors call failure to thrive—then he or she should consider testing for levels of HGH.

Quality-of-Life Assessment of
Human Growth Hormone Deficiency

	Yes	*No*
I have to struggle to finish things.	☐	☐
I feel like I've got to sleep during the day.	☐	☐
I feel lonely even when I am with other people.	☐	☐
I have to read things several times before they sink in.	☐	☐
It takes a lot of effort for me to do even the simplest of jobs.	☐	☐
I have trouble controlling my emotions.	☐	☐
I often lose my train of thought.	☐	☐
I lack confidence.	☐	☐
I've got to push myself to do things.	☐	☐
I often feel very tense.	☐	☐
I feel like I let people down.	☐	☐
I find it hard to mix with people.	☐	☐
I feel exhausted when I haven't done anything.	☐	☐
There are times when I feel very low.	☐	☐
I avoid any responsibilities.	☐	☐
I avoid socializing with people I don't know well.	☐	☐
I feel like I'm a burden.	☐	☐
I often forget what people say to me.	☐	☐
I find it hard to plan ahead.	☐	☐
I am easily irritated by people.	☐	☐
I often feel too tired to do the things I have to do.	☐	☐
I have to force myself to do everything that has to be done.	☐	☐
I often have to force myself to stay awake.	☐	☐
I have trouble remembering things.	☐	☐

Total # of Yes's_____ Total # of No's_____

Is There Anything I Can Do If My HGH Levels Are Low?

First of all, I should say that far fewer people suffer from a low HGH than hypothyroidism. As already discussed, 10 million Americans have been diagnosed with thyroid problems while a projected 50 million go undiagnosed. Fifty thousand people in the United States have been diagnosed with HGH deficiency and six thousand new cases are reported each year.

However, from what I see at my program, especially regarding obese clients, these HGH statistics should be much higher. And keep in mind that all of us will likely experience a decline in HGH as we age. It's part of the natural aging process.

For most of us, especially those with a significant HGH deficiency, we are really talking about a quality-of-life issue. The real issues are slowing the drop in HGH as you age and increasing levels if they are already low. The prescription is the Fat-Burning Metabolic Fitness Plan.

In recent years a significant number of studies have shown that specific types of exercises done at specific levels of intensity significantly increase the amount of HGH in the body. A recent report in the *Exercise and Sport Sciences Reviews* clearly shows that both aerobic exercise and resistance exercise increase HGH. An article in the *Strength and Conditioning Journal* stresses the effectiveness of interval training in stimulating the production of HGH. These are exactly the types of exercises I prescribe in my four-week program.

I have found that the most important thing to keep in mind is that you should never focus on just one particular hormone but always look at the whole picture. The body's hormonal system is like a symphony. You can't just look at estrogen or testosterone or T3 levels or HGH levels. All of these hormones are interconnected and the body needs all of them to be balanced.

7

Assess Your Stress, Burn Your Fat

We encounter stress every day—during traffic jams on the freeway, in the workplace, at home with the spouse and kids, on the evening news. We feel stress when we worry about money or retirement or whether we will get a promotion. Those of us who are middle-aged might face the stress of properly caring for aging or sick parents and our kids leaving the nest. Since September 11, we must also contend with the stress of knowing that our country and loved ones are not immune from possible terrorist attacks. Stressors surround us at every turn.

Why Do We Feel Stress?

If stress is so bad for us, then why have our bodies developed the stress response in the first place? From an evolutionary standpoint, stress is not only useful but necessary for survival. For the first two hundred thousand years of humanity's existence, stress was a useful mechanism that got our ancestors physically prepared to kill wild animals for food, run for their lives, fight an opponent, or survive a natural disaster such as a flash flood. Greater physical strength from the adrenaline rush, sharper hearing and vision, heightened brain function, and more energy to fight or flee were certainly useful.

But the catch is that stress was never meant to be a long-term condition of daily life. Our ancestors experienced the heightened physical and hormonal response of a stress reaction during times of genuine physical danger. They then discharged their energy while dealing with the problem, cleared the stress hormones out of their system, and returned to a physiologically normal state.

In the modern world, unless we are being robbed at gunpoint in a dark alley, most of our stress is psychological in nature. Therefore, it is difficult to make it go away by an immediate physical response or action that discharges it. When you discover that your new secretary has gotten your mailing lists mixed up, yelling at him or her and pounding on the desk in frustration will not solve anything.

Stress Can Make You Fat

Stress has become a condition in which we accept a short-term level of heightened performance at the expense of long-term health. Whether physical or emotional, stress has many negative effects on the body. One of them is the accumulation of a hormone called cortisol. When faced with a stressful situation, the body produces an adrenaline rush that releases fat and glucose as an energy source to help deal with the stressor. Once the crisis subsides, cortisol becomes active and stimulates the appetite so that we can replenish our fat stores. Since most of us don't reach for an apple or a chicken breast when we feel hungry, the release of cortisol usually leads to grabbing a quick carbohydrate snack such as a slice of pizza, a donut, a candy bar, or some type of high-carbohydrate fast food. Unfortunately, living with a high level of daily stress causes the body to produce a consistently high level of cortisol, leading to a vicious cycle of stress, frequent overeating, and fat gain.

Stress Weakens the Immune System

One of the more serious effects of stress is that it redirects metabolic energy away from the immune system. A tremendous amount of energy is necessary to operate the complex cells, hormones, and organs that make up this system. Fifteen minutes of danger and a return to normal isn't going to compromise your immune system, but living with constant stress will surely slow you down metabolically, making you more susceptible to illness. Stress can lead to stroke, hypertension, and type 2 diabetes. In fact, the six leading causes of death in the United States—heart disease, cancer, lung ailments, accidents, cirrhosis of the liver, and suicide—are directly related to stress.

One recent study of how chronic stress weakens the immune system found that the protein interleukin-6 (IL-6) was present in unusually high amounts in people who suffered from chronic stress. IL-6 normally triggers inflammation to help fight infections. It also stimulates the production of C-reactive protein, which is a very accurate predictor of heart attack risk. High levels of IL-6 are also associated with type 2 diabetes, some cancers, osteoporosis, arthritis, and depression. Prolonged high levels of IL-6 can lead to a syndrome called permanently aged immune response.

This study also showed that very simple lifestyle changes, such as getting enough sleep, eating properly, stopping smoking, and exercising regularly, can dramatically reduce levels of IL-6.

How Stressed Are You?

Since all of us are stressed at one time or another, it is important to differentiate between being able to handle stress and feeling overstressed. I have written extensively about stress self-evaluation and stress management in *Maximum Energy for Life,* and I refer you to that book if you feel that not being able to handle stress is a major problem in your life. An important point to remember is that you will never be able to get rid of all of the stress in your life. The real goals should be learning to get rid of unnecessary stress by making wiser lifestyle, work, and relationship decisions and learning how to manage the stress you can't avoid.

This chapter has two simple questionnaires on stress and depression designed by the National Mental Health Association (NMHA). Some of their tips for controlling stress are also included.

NMHA Stress Checklist

Everyone handles stress differently—some better than others. If you think you have too much stress in your life, it may be helpful to talk with a doctor, clergy member, or other caring professional. Because reactions to stress can be a factor in depression, anxiety, and other mental and emotional disorders, you may consider working with a psychiatrist, psychologist, social worker, or other qualified counselor.

Checklist of Negative Reactions to Stress and Tension

	Yes	No
1. Do minor problems and disappointments upset you excessively?	☐	☐
2. Are you unable to stop worrying?	☐	☐

3. Do you feel inadequate or suffer from self-doubt?   ☐   ☐
4. Are you constantly tired?   ☐   ☐
5. Do you experience flashes of anger over minor problems?   ☐   ☐
6. Have you noticed a change in sleeping or eating patterns?   ☐   ☐
7. Do you suffer from chronic pain, headaches, or backaches?   ☐   ☐

If you answered yes to most of these questions, consider the following suggestions for reducing or controlling stress:

- *Be realistic.* If you feel overwhelmed by some activities, learn to say no!
- *Shed the superman/superwoman urge.* No one is perfect, so don't expect perfection from yourself or others.
- *Meditate* for ten to twenty minutes a day.
- *Visualize* how you can manage a stressful situation more successfully.
- *Take one thing at a time.* Prioritize your tasks and tackle each one separately.
- *Find a hobby* that will give you a break from your worries.
- *Live a healthy lifestyle* with good nutrition, adequate rest, regular exercise, limited caffeine and alcohol, and balanced work and play.
- *Share your feelings* with family and friends. Don't try to cope alone.
- *Give in occasionally.* Be flexible.
- *Go easy with criticism.* You may be expecting too much.

NMHA Depression Checklist

Every year more than 19 million Americans experience clinical depression. It affects men, women, and children of all races and socioeconomic groups, causing them to lose motivation, energy, and the pleasure of everyday life. Clinical depression often goes untreated because people don't recognize many of its symptoms. The good news is that almost everyone who gets treated can soon feel better.

Here is a checklist of ten symptoms of clinical depression:

- A persistent sad, anxious, or "empty" mood
- Sleeping too little or sleeping too much

- Reduced appetite and weight loss or increased appetite and weight gain
- Loss of interest or pleasure in activities once enjoyed
- Restlessness or irritability
- Persistent physical symptoms that don't respond to treatment (such as headaches, chronic pain, or constipation and other digestive disorders)
- Difficulty concentrating, remembering, or making decisions
- Fatigue or loss of energy
- Feeling guilty, hopeless, or worthless
- Thoughts of death or suicide

If you experience five or more of these symptoms for longer than two weeks, or if the symptoms are severe enough to interfere with your daily routine, see your doctor or a qualified mental health professional.

For more information on depression, or to locate a free, confidential, and professional depression screening site in your area, call the National Mental Health Association at 800-969-NMHA (6642) or visit www.nmha.org for a confidential online depression screening.

The Rahe Life Stress Scale

Another helpful resource for evaluating stress levels is the well-known Rahe Life Stress Scale developed by Dr. Thomas Holmes and Dr. Richard H. Rahe, researchers at the University of Washington School of Medicine in Seattle. Based on their years of researching the connection between stress and health, these doctors have assigned numerical values to stressful events. For example, the death of a spouse is 119 points, pregnancy is 67, divorce is 96, changing jobs is 51, and sexual difficulties are 44. Even events that you might think of as good or pleasurable have an impact on your overall stress level. Marriage is 50 points, a major increase in income is 38 points, a vacation is 24, and the birth of a grandchild is 43. According to Drs. Holmes and Rahe, if you score below 200, you have only a low risk of illness. Between 201 and 300, your chances of getting sick are moderate. A score between 301 and 450 increases your odds of getting sick considerably, and a score greater than 450 puts you at imminent risk. While this test is not an absolute indicator of your risk for disease, it can give you a clearer picture of how many of your daily life circumstances are potentially stressful. If you wish to take this test, you can access it on the Internet at Dr. Rahe's Web site: www.hapi-health.com.

Three Strategies for Combating Stress

Strategy #1: Learn the Benefits of Good Nutrition on Stress

If a healthy person is fasting or starving, 90 percent of his or her calories will come from fat stores and only 10 percent from protein. When a person is undergoing chronic stress, even if he or she is not injured or sick, only 70 percent of calories will come from fat stores and 30 percent will come from lean protein.

There is a direct correlation between the breakdown of protein for fuel and the greater metabolic need for glucose during times of physical or emotional stress or trauma. To get the extra glucose, the body takes amino acids from lean muscle mass, converts them to alanine, and changes the alanine into glucose to be used by the tissues as an emergency energy supply. Physiological stress can greatly increase metabolic requirements. For example, after surgery metabolic needs increase by 20 percent; following a serious infection or a traumatic injury, they increase by 50 percent.

Following a well-balanced and nutritional diet such as the Fat-Burning Metabolic Fitness Nutritional Plan becomes even more crucial when you are suffering from the effects of illness or long-term stress.

Strategy #2: Exercise to Reduce Stress

People who live with high levels of stress will be amazed at how effectively exercise combats stress. Stress is a killer because it undermines almost every system in the body, from the cardiovascular system to the immune system. Since I work with so many professionals whose jobs come with an unavoidable stress component, I am always gratified to see how greatly my Fat-Burning Metabolic Fitness Exercise Plan improves their ability to handle stress.

Bo Walker, the radio host who agreed to participate in a makeover for *Let's Live* magazine, worked very hard at my plan and kept exercising even when the twelve-week makeover period was completed and the magazine articles had gone to press. Bo's moment of truth came when the radio station announced that they were not renewing his contract. Suddenly, he was faced with the stress of being the forty-year-old unemployed father of a two-year-old child with financial, career, and self-esteem issues.

Once his job had officially ended, Bo felt no motivation at all to go to the gym. But his wife, Lisa, told him, "You've got to continue doing this for your own sanity." Not giving up on his exercise program turned out to be Bo's greatest emotional stabilizer: "It kept my mind occupied. I knew I had someplace to go two, three days out of the week. The exercise was cathartic. It allowed me to keep my mind off losing my job. It did more than just make me feel physically better. It was an emotional boost as well. Once I was at the gym, I could do my routine. It put me back on the track again. It's helped me through quite a bit."

Fortunately, Bo was only out of work for a few months. Sticking with his exercise program gave him the ability to reduce his stress and have the energy and focus he needed to find another job and get on with his life.

The two forms of exercise offered in the Fat-Burning Metabolic Fitness Exercise Plan are specifically designed to deal with stress. If you must navigate a series of several stressful events daily, then the steady-state exercises on days 1, 3, and 5 will help to create greater emotional homeostasis so that you can cope better. If you are experiencing continuous stress, such as having to be the caregiver for someone in the family who is seriously ill, the core and interval exercises on days 2, 4, and 6 will enable you to achieve greater emotional and physical equilibrium.

Strategy #3: Learn Gender-Specific Stress-Fighting Techniques

In 1994, the National Institute of Health mandated that both genders be more equally represented in the studies done by government and other medical research groups. One of the more interesting outcomes of that decision has been the discovery that men and women are biologically programmed to have different reactions to stress.

When a research team at UCLA led by Shelley E. Taylor analyzed hundreds of stress studies done since 1985, they discovered that men and women release different hormones during stressful situations that result in different styles of coping. Men usually respond with the classic fight-or-flight behavior, increased arousal, and greater risk taking, which for many years had been considered the accepted model for both genders. However, it is now becoming clear that women more often manage stress by seeking out bonding activities.

The mechanism behind this response is the release of the hormone oxytocin. While the large amounts of testosterone produced in men during stress tend to counteract this hormone, estrogen enhances its effect. Oxytocin buffers the fight-or-flight response in women and instead encourages them to care for children and bond with other women. "Women are more likely to seek emotional comfort and solace by calling up a friend or relative," Taylor says. These tending or befriending behaviors cause the body to release more oxytocin, producing a further calming affect.

One of my clients who was diagnosed with breast cancer spent a lot of time talking with her friends and family during her months of treatment: "Cancer is a great shock to everyone involved, not just the patient. I discovered that my relatives and friends were just as stressed as I was, and my parents and siblings really felt helpless because they lived all the way on the other side of the country. But when we kept in touch by phone and e-mail, it helped us a lot. My friends also appreciated it when I told them how I was really feeling and what I needed. It helped them to cope with their fear and anxiety. Letting them comfort me or bring over some food made them feel calmer and more empowered because they were doing something for me."

Another gender difference is that women tend to feel more day-to-day stress than men. The reasons for this can be seen in how women's emotional lives are structured.

- Women engage in more multitasking than men in their everyday lives. A man may be the father and breadwinner, but a woman is the mother, career woman, housekeeper, caretaker, and friend and supporter of many other women. All of these activities take their toll, creating greater stress.
- Women are more vulnerable to physical violence, mugging, and rape than men.
- For a woman to be happy, she has to be in a good relationship with all of the people who are important to her including her kids, her spouse, her family, her coworkers, and her friends.
- Women are programmed to nurture, caretake, and defer to others, most often at the expense of their own emotional needs.
- Because nature designed women for child rearing, they are naturally hardwired to be more sensitive to their environment than men.

Stress Tips for Women

1. Get enough sleep at night.
2. Don't skip meals. Have three square meals a day and two snacks.
3. Exercise regularly and at appropriate intensity levels for your gender. (See chapters 12 and 13.)
4. Practice meditation or deep-breathing exercises for at least ten minutes a day.

5. Make time for yourself. Take a relaxing aromatherapy bath; listen to music; take a walk in a beautiful setting; do some gardening; buy yourself roses.
6. Try to be conscious of your needs and don't always put yourself last.

Stress Tips for Men

1. Get enough sleep at night.
2. Don't skip meals. Have three square meals a day and two snacks.
3. Exercise regularly and at appropriate intensity levels for your gender. (See chapters 12 and 13.)
4. Take up a recreational sport to help alleviate competitional stresses in the workplace.
5. Do yoga to help dissipate the effects of continual muscle contraction. Men tend to have greater continual contraction than women of the fight-or-flight muscles and they need to elongate them.
6. Learn to walk through your fears. For example, take a public speaking course or a self-esteem workshop.

PART TWO

The Fat-Burning Metabolic Fitness Nutritional Plan

8

Increase Your Metabolism and Burn Fat

Food Programming versus Dieting

I am often surprised at how little people understand about how the three food groups—proteins, carbohydrates, and fats—function in synergy to maintain physical health. You cannot avoid consuming any one of these kinds of nutrients and expect to be slim, metabolically efficient, and balanced. Yet we live in a culture where popular diet books have made fats and/or carbohydrates the foods to avoid. Some diet gurus advocate an almost total avoidance of carbohydrates and a large intake of protein. Others give you the idea that all fats are bad—the eating-fats-equals-getting-fat myth. And some downplay the importance of choosing unsaturated fats, such as olive oil and soy butter, over saturated fats, such as dairy butter and cheese, telling you that it is actually healthy to eat foods with lots of butter and cream sauces. Of course, these foods taste good, but is a constant diet of foods cooked in butter, covered with melted cheese, and swimming in cream sauce good for you?

The bottom line is that over the short term you can probably lose weight on almost any diet out there, no matter how strange or how calorically restrictive. But you should ask the following questions when considering a new food program:

- Will this program work in the long run? In other words, will you be able to keep the fat off once you've managed to take it off?

- Is this program so calorically restrictive that you will have to live with hunger 24/7 (and be tempted to go off your diet or binge)?
- Will this program help you lose body fat while rebuilding lean muscle mass?
- Will this food program make you healthier—that is, lower your cholesterol and triglycerides?
- Will this program help you feel energized or make you exhausted and cranky?

Five Key Reasons for Following This Nutritional Plan

The Fat-Burning Metabolic Fitness Nutritional Plan meets all of the criteria above, plus it is designed to support and work in tandem with the Fat-Burning Metabolic Fitness Exercise Plan to help you lose the maximum amount of fat. The duration and intensity of each exercise module in chapter 13 has been carefully planned to work in synergy with the balanced energy (caloric) deficit of my meal plans. The timing of when you eat and when you exercise is also very important. Exercising before a meal increases metabolism, elevating your fat-burning capacity even hours after the exercise is over. This is known as the thermic effect of food. For example, a recent article in the *International Journal of Sport Nutrition and Exercise Metabolism* shows how resistive exercise enhances the body's ability to metabolize foods, especially carbohydrates. Cardiovascular exercise, when done at the proper intensity for the proper amount of time, has the same effect. See chapter 12 for a thorough discussion of how this works.

There are five key reasons why my food plan not only takes off the fat but helps you to stay slim over the long run.

1. It is intelligently balanced between proteins, carbohydrates, and fats based on the evidence presented by nutritional science.
2. It will adequately satisfy your body's daily caloric requirements.
3. This program never puts your daily caloric intake so low that you will feel undue hunger, physical or emotional stress, or loss of energy.
4. It provides you with three balanced meals and two snacks per day to keep your energy levels consistent.
5. Since we are all a bit different from one another, it has a certain amount of flexibility built into it to allow for your individual nutri-

tional needs. For example, a man or a woman who is very athletic will require more protein than someone who is more sedentary.

Eat the Right Percentages of Protein, Carbohydrates, and Fats

The latest research shows that 30 percent lean protein, 40 percent low-glycemic carbohydrates, and 30 percent acceptable fats work best for metabolic efficiency. These percentages have been tremendously effective in my program for athletes who want to lose fat, build more lean muscle, and improve performance, and for people who are overfat and often suffering from either elevated triglycerides or high glucose levels. A recent article in the *American Journal of Clinical Nutrition* makes a convincing argument for this ratio in people suffering from type 2 diabetes, stating that eating 30 percent dietary protein and 40 percent carbohydrates appears to improve glycemic control without increasing the risk of heart disease. In as little as five weeks, the glucose levels of the study participants dropped an astonishing 40 percent, and blood lipids, especially triglycerides, were significantly lowered.

Now let's take a look at the three food groups and the role each nutrient plays in the body.

Proteins

I suggest a daily intake of 30 percent lean protein. Good sources of protein are chicken breasts, all types of fish, beef with a low fat content (in moderation), soy products, and whey products. Protein is a stabilizing food that assists in insulin management, the building of lean muscle, and immune function. For men, ingesting adequate amounts of protein daily helps stop the decrease in testosterone levels that they experience as they age. An article in the *Journal of Clinical Endocrinology and Metabolism* states, "Diets low in protein lead to increases in sex hormone–binding globulin in older men, potentially reducing the availability of testosterone and causing loss of muscle mass, red cell mass and bone density." Getting adequate protein also helps avoid or slow bone loss in women, especially after menopause.

Because protein is not stored, three balanced meals and two or three snacks per day that include protein are required to suppress hunger and burn body fat during physical exercise. When choosing protein sources, always choose lean meats and low-fat dairy. First-choice protein sources include skim milk; fat-free cheese and cottage cheese; yogurt made from skim milk; 95 percent lean ground beef, turkey, or encased meats (sausage, bologna, etc.); skinless chicken breasts; white-meat tuna in water; egg whites; and nonfried fish and seafood.

I always suggest that clients eat cold-water fish such as salmon and halibut at least twice a week, or even once daily if they really love fish. According to the *American Journal of Clinical Nutrition,* eating fish daily decreases insulin levels, increases glucose production, lowers triglyceride (bad fat) production, and increases the level of HDL (good) cholesterol, reducing your risk of cardiovascular disease.

Many people are concerned about the dangers of mercury in fish. This is something you should pay heed to, especially if you are pregnant or nursing, or if you have children in your family. Generally, you should avoid eating swordfish, tilefish, and king mackerel more than once a week, since these larger oceangoing fish have accumulated larger concentrations of mercury in their bodies. When it comes to tuna, the type that has the highest level of mercury is albacore. Therefore, if you want to give your family a tuna fish sandwich, choose light tuna, which has very low mercury concentrations. Freshwater mackerel, cod, and sardines are also safe bets.

Another tip that can help lessen your risk of mercury exposure is to eat several tropical fruits every week. Mangoes, bananas, pineapples, and papayas may help to reduce the amount of mercury that your body absorbs. When a study was made of a group of women from a predominantly fish-eating community, it was discovered that those who ate the largest amount of tropical fruits had the lowest mercury levels.

Soy

Soy products have always been a part of my nutritional programs because of their many benefits. Research studies have shown that an overabundance of the amino acid lysine increases the level of bad cholesterol in the body, while the amino acid arginine decreases it. Compared to animal protein, soy has a more favorable ratio of arginine to lysine. This lower ratio decreases the body's production of insulin and increases its production of glucagon. So, eating soy frequently helps you shift your metabolism from fat storage to fat mobilization.

Soy products may also lower the risk of coronary disease. And when used in conjunction with a properly balanced nutrition and aerobic exercise program, they are an important tool for lowering your body fat and cholesterol levels. Studies have shown that soy foods also lower the risk of hormone-related cancers.

Besides soy-based powders, there are many delicious soy food products available, including soy burgers and hot dogs, as well as many varieties of tofu, soy cheeses, and soy milk. Since one of the challenges faced by vegetarians is getting sufficient protein in their daily diet, soy products can be a nutritional mainstay.

Whey Protein Powder: The Perfect Between-Meal Snack

I encourage my clients and the professional athletes with whom I work to drink a whey protein shake as a snack between meals. I also recommend that all of my clients have a whey protein drink immediately before doing resistance exercise. The reason is twofold: to decrease the amount of muscle tissue broken down during an exercise session and to aid in the synthesis of protein as muscles are being rebuilt and strengthened. A recent article in the *Exercise and Sport Sciences Reviews* states that ingesting foods (such as whey powder) that contain both carbohydrates and amino acid–rich proteins causes "a substantial increase in muscle protein synthesis and a lesser inhibition of muscle protein breakdown, the net result being an increase in muscle protein accretion."

A wide range of excellent whey powders is available in health food stores. Rich in glutamine and essential amino acids, whey protein is a superior protein choice for many reasons.

- Whey stimulates the metabolism. The amino acid profile of whey enhances recovery from exercise by stimulating muscle protein synthesis.
- Whey is derived from calcium-rich milk products. Foods with a high calcium content increase fat loss, especially if you are on a low-calorie diet.
- Whey helps the body to recover more quickly from the stress of exercise.
- Whey gives strong support to the immune system.
- Due to its high amino acid and glutamine content, whey supports gastrointestinal health and offers relief from digestive distress such as cramps, bloating, and diarrhea.
- Two major proteins in whey, lactoferrin and lactoferricin, function as antioxidants due to their iron-binding capacity. Whey also contains cysteine-rich proteins, which are pivotal in the synthesis of glutathione, a major intercellular antioxidant.

Always read the label carefully and avoid brands with higher amounts of sugar. One excellent product is American Whey Protein by Jarrow, which has 18 grams of protein and 3.7 grams of glutamine per scoop. You can purchase this product at a local health food store or on the Internet.

Carbohydrates

I suggest 40 percent low-glycemic, complex carbohydrates. Some clients find that amount of carbs intimidating because many popular diet books have caused people to shift their dietary fears from fats to carbohydrates. The key is to learn how to manage your intake of carbs relative to your activity level. While people can lose pounds of scale weight on a low-carbohydrate diet, it's a sure thing that they will feel irritable, headachy, and fatigued. To maintain the brain and central nervous system, the body needs a certain amount of glucose, which it gets from sugars and starches, the by-products of carbohydrates after digestion. This glucose is stored in the liver and in the muscles. When you do not eat a sufficient amount of carbohydrates daily, your body has to get its supply from somewhere. At that point, it will begin breaking down its own muscle protein to synthesize glucose to adequately supply vital organs. So, the weight you are losing on a low-carbohydrate diet will be muscle tissue, not fat, because your body cannot break down its fat stores into glucogen.

The goal of any good weight-loss program should always be to lose as little muscle as possible. For every gram of muscle tissue you lose, you lose 4 grams of water; but for every gram of fat, you lose only 1 gram of water. Water weight is not true long-term weight loss because water is the easiest thing in the world to gain back. After losing weight on a diet, if you begin eating a normal amount of carbohydrates—or, if you are the average American, an excessive amount of carbohydrates—your body will quickly regain its lost muscle tissue and its associated water weight.

The goal of my Fat-Burning Metabolic Fitness Plan is to spare your lean muscle tissue while you lose the maximum amount of fat. Since a pound of fat is roughly three times the volume of a pound of lean muscle, losing pounds of fat will create the greatest transformation in your physical appearance. So, do not be afraid of eating 40 percent carbohydrates. The key is to eat the right kinds of carbohydrates.

What Is the "Right" Kind of Carbohydrate?

An important criterion to keep in mind when choosing appropriate carbohydrates is their rating on the Glycemic Index. Foods with a high glycemic rating stimulate a higher than normal production of insulin and tend to stimulate fat storage. Foods that have a low glycemic rating do not significantly elevate insulin or stimulate fat storage. High-glycemic foods should be avoided or eaten in moderation.

Eating low-glycemic foods is especially important if you suffer from type 1 or type 2 diabetes. A recent study conducted by the University of Sydney, Australia, and published in *Diabetes Care* analyzed the results of fourteen different studies around the world to see if eating low-glycemic foods really benefited diabetics. When the results were compiled, they showed a clear improvement in levels of glucose in the study participants.

All foods have a glycemic index, but when it comes to carbohydrates, you can think of them in terms of simple (high-glycemic carbs) and complex (low-glycemic carbs). Examples of simple carbohydrates are potatoes, white bread, bananas, white rice, pancakes, desserts, sugary soft drinks, pizza, french fries, and candy. Examples of complex carbohydrates include yams, sweet potatoes, brown rice, whole-grain cereals, bran or flaxseed muffins, apples, and oatmeal. For a more extensive list of high- and low-glycemic index foods, see my book *Lose Your Love Handles.*

Eat at Least Five Fruits and Vegetables a Day

Many of you have heard of the U.S. Department of Health's Five-a-Day Campaign that is aimed at helping Americans to be healthier. Fruits and vegetables—low in calories and packed with vitamins, minerals, and fiber—are vital to a healthy diet. The DOH has shown that increasing your daily consumption of vegetables and fruits in a rainbow assortment of colors could decrease early deaths from our nation's two biggest killers, cancer and coronary heart disease, by 20 percent and 40 percent, respectively.

Blue or purple fruits and vegetables, which contain varying amounts of health-promoting phytochemicals such as anthocyanins and phenolics, have antioxidant and antiaging benefits, promote memory function, and lower the risk for certain types of cancers. Foods in the blue/purple category include blackberries, blueberries, plums, purple figs, purple grapes, purple cabbage, eggplant, and purple-fleshed potatoes.

Green fruits and vegetables contain varying amounts of potent phytochemicals such as lutein and indoles, which have antioxidant and other health-promoting benefits such as creating stronger bones, promoting keener vision, and helping to prevent cancer. Foods in the green category include avocados, green apples, green grapes, honeydew, kiwifruit, limes, artichokes, arugula, asparagus, broccoli, brussels sprouts, green beans, green cabbage, celery, cucumbers, endive, leafy greens, lettuce, green onions, peas, and spinach.

White, tan, and brown fruits and vegetables contain varying amounts of phytochemicals that help to maintain good levels of cholesterol, promote heart health, and prevent some kinds of cancers such as breast cancer. This category includes brown pears, white nectarines, white peaches, cauliflower, garlic, ginger, mushrooms, onions, white-fleshed potatoes, shallots, and turnips.

Orange and yellow fruits and vegetables contain varying amounts of antioxidants such as vitamin C, as well as carotenoids and bioflavonoids, two classes of phytochemicals that promote health. Eating these kinds of foods will contribute to your having a healthy heart, healthy vision, strong immune function, and lowered risk of some types of cancers. Orange and yellow fruits and vegetables include yellow apples, apricots, cantaloupe, grapefruit, lemons, mangoes, nectarines, oranges, papayas, peaches, yellow pears, tangerines, yellow beets, butternut squash, carrots, yellow peppers, yellow potatoes, yellow summer squash, yellow winter squash, sweet potatoes, and yellow tomatoes.

Red fruits and vegetables promote a healthy urinary tract, heart health, and good memory function and protect against certain types of cancers. These foods include red apples, blood oranges, cherries, cranberries, red grapes, pink/red grapefruit, red pears, raspberries, strawberries, watermelon, beets, red peppers, radishes, radicchio, red onions, red potatoes, rhubarb, and tomatoes.

Fruits and Vegetables Decrease Bone Loss and Lower Blood Pressure

A September 2003 Medscape article showed the importance of fruits and vegetables in combating hypertension and bone loss due to aging and poor nutritional health. A recent study conducted by DASH (Dietary Approaches to Stopping Hypertension) showed that a diet rich in fruit and vegetables was associated with a significant fall in blood pressure. Increasing fruit and vegetable intake from 3.6 to 9.5 servings daily also decreased the amount of urinary calcium that subjects excreted by close to 50 percent. While some researchers suggested that this was due to the "high fiber content of the diet possibly impeding calcium absorption," others claimed that a more likely explanation was a reduction in the body's "acid load." If you can maintain a good level of alkalinity in your body, which fruits and vegetables provide in abundance, you will excrete less calcium. As people get older, their bodies become more acidic. Therefore, eating the proper amount of fruits and vegetables every day can guard against developing osteoporosis.

Another element found in fruits and vegetables that promotes healthy bones is potassium. A wide spectrum of population-based studies published between 2001 and 2003 showed the beneficial effect of fruit and vegetable/potassium intake on the bone health of people of all ages.

Fats

Many of my clients have the mistaken notion that if they avoid eating fats, they won't get fat. Most people do not realize that fats are a wonderful source of energy, and many fats, like fish or fish oils containing omega-3, can lower cholesterol, improve joint health, and help protect against cancer. Ingesting a daily diet of 30 percent of the right kinds of fats actually enables you to utilize dietary fat to help burn body fat. The reason is that all fats produce 9 calories of energy per gram, and the body uses fats mostly as an energy source, along with glucose broken down from the digestion of carbohydrates.

There are three different groups of fats: saturated fats, trans fatty acids, and monounsaturated fats.

Saturated fats should only be eaten in limited amounts because they can raise your cholesterol, increasing your chances of heart disease. People who eat diets high in saturated fats also run a greater risk of developing diabetes and some kinds of cancers. These types of fats are found in meat and dairy products such as beef, pork, cheese, and butter.

Trans fatty acids pose an even greater threat to your cholesterol and heart health. Studies have shown that eating too much of them increases your risk of developing diabetes even more than eating saturated fats. Trans fatty acids are formed when either vegetables or fish oils are hydrogenated. French fries, donuts, cookies, chips, and other snack foods are all high in trans fatty acids. In fact, nearly all fried or baked goods have some trans fat content.

The best kind of fat to include in your daily diet is monounsaturated fat, which is found in plant products such as vegetable oils, nuts, and avocados. Your body uses this type of fat to strengthen cell membranes, support nerve and hormone function, and produce hormone-like substances called prostaglandins, which have been linked to the prevention of heart disease and cancers.

Essential Fatty Acids Decrease Health Risks

Two kinds of unsaturated fats are necessary for your survival. These are the essential fatty acids omega-6 (linoleic acid) and omega-3 (linolenic acid). Since your body cannot manufacture these fatty acids, they must be obtained from the foods you eat. Omega-6 is fairly common and is found in most vegetable oils. Keep in mind that it is probably better to buy your oils in amber or green bottles, since exposure to sunlight destroys freshness and can turn oils rancid. It is also better to buy them in health food stores if you can. Most typical grocery store oils, which are processed for mass distribution, are often filled with free radicals—that is, substances that can damage cells—and trans fatty acids.

Omega-3 is found in soy, walnut, flax, fish, and canola oils and in dark green, leafy vegetables. It is especially important to make sure that you supplement your food plan with enough omega-3 fats, since the American diet is usually deficient in this nutrient. Any doctor who treats cancer patients will suggest getting an adequate amount of omega-3 in the diet because it is a great protector from many types of cancers, especially breast cancer. While the ideal ratio of omega-6 to omega-3 should be between 3:1 and 4:1, a recent study showed that most people have twenty times the level of omega-6 than omega-3.

The Nine Benefits of "Good" Fats

There are many benefits to eating the proper amounts of unsaturated fats and essential fatty acids.

1. They decrease free radicals in the body.
2. They lower total cholesterol levels by preventing platelet aggregation and vasoconstriction.
3. Good fats lower triglycerides.
4. They raise levels of HDL.
5. Good fats lower blood pressure.
6. They decrease symptoms of heart palpitations, also known as angina.
7. They lower the risk of heart attacks and strokes.
8. They decrease the pain and swelling of rheumatoid arthritis.
9. Good fats lower the risk for many types of cancers including breast cancer.

How to Increase the Essential Fatty Acids in Your Diet

There are several other ways to increase the amount of essential fatty acids in your diet. For example, cold-water fish such as salmon, mackerel, and trout are rich sources of the essential fatty acid metabolites DHA (docosahexaenoic acid) and EPA (eicosapentaenoic acid). These have been shown to help lower blood pressure, improve cholesterol levels, and lower risk for cardiovascular disease. Aside from eating fish a minimum of twice per week, you can supplement your diet with omega-3 by taking fish oil capsules, which are available at most pharmacies and health food stores.

Much research has been done across gender lines to ascertain whether essential fatty acids can benefit men and women who are experiencing the changes associated with midlife. A recent study published in *Circulation* studied a group of middle-aged men who had never experienced coronary heart disease. The common link they found was frequent consumption of fish. The more fish the men ate per week, the lower their cholesterol, triglycerides, blood pressure, and heart rate. Since researchers have found that even small reductions in heart rate can have a significant impact on cardiovascular health, eating fish at least twice a week is a simple way to minimize or avoid heart disease. The famous U.S. Physicians Health Study, which followed 20,551 male doctors for eleven years, found that individuals who ate fish at least once a week had a 52 percent lower incidence of sudden cardiac death than men who did not eat fish.

Getting enough omega-3 by eating fish also has health benefits for women. The famous Nurses Health Study, which followed 84,000 nurses over sixteen years, showed that the more fish the women ate weekly, the lower their risk for cardiovascular disease. An article published in the *Journal of Nutritional Biochemistry* showed that eating fish or taking fish oil supplements lowered cholesterol and triglycerides and decreased inflammatory markers (markers for heart attack) in postmenopausal women who were using some sort of hormone replacement therapy, and it actually reversed some of the undesirable risk factors for heart disease caused by HRT. This is especially significant since a woman's risk for heart disease after menopause becomes equal to a man's.

Flax oil is another rich source of omega-3 and all other essential fatty acids, which is why bodybuilders often mix it into their protein drinks. It is best taken not in capsules but in liquid form to assure freshness and quality. The next time you are fixing a green salad, try using a tablespoon of flax oil as a dressing, or half a tablespoon mixed with sunflower oil or a little vinegar. You may also lightly brush it over meat after it has been cooked. Mixing flax oil with low-fat cottage cheese helps your body to utilize it, since the sulfur content of cottage cheese enhances the effectiveness of the oil. Ground flaxseed, which you can sprinkle over your breakfast cereal or your salad, add to baked bread or muffins, or blend into a protein drink, is another great source of omega-3.

Other Sources of Unsaturated Fats
Other acceptable sources of unsaturated fats include Hellmann's Light
Mayonnaise, Kraft Light Mayonnaise, Smart Balance Soft Spread (no
trans fatty acids), and unsaturated corn oil. Products such as Promise, Take
Control, Fleischmann's Margarine, and I Can't Believe It's Not Butter
(spray, not solid) are excellent butter alternatives. If real butter is your only
alternative when dining out, use it in moderation.

Fiber Is Important

Fiber is simply plant food that passes undigested through the small intes-
tine. There are two basic types of fiber: insoluble and soluble. Insoluble
fiber holds less water and includes vegetables, most bran products, and
whole grains. These food types provide bulk and help to normalize bowel
movements. Soluble fibers hold up to forty times their weight in water and
include oats, any type of legume, beans, and psyllium. Citrus and apples,
the most soluble fibers, hold one hundred times their weight in water.

These items provide the primary food source for friendly bacteria in the
intestinal track. When you do not get enough soluble fiber in your daily diet,
this can lead to reduced growth of friendly bacteria, increased growth of
unfriendly bacteria, constipation, and increased risk for colorectal cancer.

The National Cancer Institute and the American Heart Association
recommend eating an average of 25 to 30 grams daily. A recent study published in the *Archives of Internal Medicine* shows that a high intake of
dietary fiber, especially water-soluble fiber, is associated with a reduction
of coronary heart disease.

If you have type 1 or type 2 diabetes, eating twice the recommended
amount of fiber can have a significant effect on your blood sugar levels. A
study by the American Diabetes Association indicates that diabetics could
significantly reduce their blood sugar by eating up to 50 grams of fiber per
day. This study also showed that a high-fiber diet improved cholesterol
levels and lowered the participants' risk of heart disease, which is a major
cause of death among people with diabetes.

A long-term study published recently in the *Journal of the American
Medical Association* stated that eating a high-fiber diet also helps to take
off the fat and keep it off. Young adults who ate at least 21 grams of fiber
per day gained an average of 8 pounds less over a ten-year period than
those who ate the least amount of fiber. When you consider that a bowl of
oatmeal or whole-grain cereal can contain up to 25 grams of fiber, it is not
difficult to get sufficient fiber in your daily diet.

High-fiber foods include the following:

- Raw or lightly cooked vegetables
- Cereals, rolls, and bread made from whole-grain flour
- Nuts, beans, peas, lentils, potatoes, and yams (with the skins on)
- Whole grains, such as whole wheat, brown rice, whole or rolled oats, buckwheat, amaranth, and brown rice
- Raw fruits such as apples (with the skins on) and oranges
- Dried fruits such as raisins, apricots, dates, and prunes (Buy organic dried fruits, since the drying process concentrates the level of fungicides and pesticides.)

When you increase your daily intake of fiber, do it slowly at first to avoid discomfort and flatulence. Make sure to take a multivitamin, since fiber speeds digestion and might deplete the body of certain vitamins.

Save Your Life

Good nutrition will help you to lose body fat and build lean muscle. But there is another side to the story. Eating properly can often mean the difference between good health and poor health—and even between life and death.

I have learned that there is no way that you can underestimate the healing power of good nutrition. A client of mine was diagnosed with breast cancer last year. This meant four months of grueling chemotherapy, recovery from surgery, and six weeks of radiation treatments. She told me that even though she sometimes had to literally force herself to eat when she had no appetite, she kept remembering what I'd taught her about good nutrition being the first line of defense against disease. She attributed her ability to be able to bounce back quickly from each of her treatments to her understanding of what supplements enhanced metabolic function and how food, especially lean protein in the form of fish and whey protein shakes, strengthened the immune system.

The other day, she gave me one of the most moving compliments I have ever received. She said, "Mackie, I think you literally saved my life. If I hadn't started your program two and a half years before I was diagnosed, I think my story would have been a lot different. My tumor was 6.5 by 8.5 centimeters. Yet it had not metastasized anywhere else in my body or even gone into my lymph nodes. At the time of my mammogram, I had never felt better or been in better shape in my entire life. I know that your program kick-started my immune system, enabling my body to fight back and save me. Most important, I feel pretty confident that I will never get cancer again because you have taught me how to eat right, exercise right, and make the right kinds of lifestyle choices for health."

Americans suffer from many illnesses that could be avoided or minimized if only they would learn to eat the proper nutrients. In the next chapter I will show you how to put all of these foods together into meal plans that will help you increase your metabolic efficiency and lose fat without ever feeling hungry.

9

Foods That Burn Fat

The science of nutrition—the beneficial effects that food has on healing and disease prevention—is receiving more and more credence in the modern medical community. In fact, a new development in the insurance industry is the assigning of special codes for the nutritional treatment of obesity, morbid obesity, and Metabolic Syndrome X.

Below are several meal plans developed by my nutritionist, Molly Kimball. (We call them Mackie Meals!) All of them are divided along the lines of 30 percent lean protein, 40 percent low-glycemic carbohydrates, and 30 percent monounsaturated fats. We have categorized them into six caloric spreads based on gender: 1,200 calories, 1,350 calories, and 1,500 calories for most women and 1,600 calories, 1,800 calories, and 2,000 calories for most men. In the case of a shorter man with a small frame or a taller woman with a large frame, there will sometimes be a caloric crossover. Also keep in mind that when you calculate your daily caloric requirements, you will not necessarily fall exactly into any one of these caloric spreads. Simply pick the plan that is closest to your number. That one will best serve your caloric needs.

You Must Exercise While You Diet

Many studies have shown that while dieting alone is effective in reducing overall weight, following a good exercise program such as the one presented in chapters 12 and 13 makes your body even more efficient at losing fat, especially during the first month of your fat-reducing program.

Ten minutes of exercise is approximately equal to 100 calories burned. The basic four-week Fat-Burning Metabolic Fitness Exercise Plan calls for 300 minutes of exercise per week, resulting in about 3,000 calories burned from physical energy expenditure alone. So, by exercise alone, you will be losing close to one pound of fat per week. The added benefit is that the program is designed so that you are exponentially increasing your metabolic rate. So, you are losing fat on three fronts: from the food plan, from the exercise plan, and from a metabolic boost.

Determine Your Caloric Needs

The best way to determine how many calories your body actually needs is by estimating your total daily caloric expenditure. This figure will include your resting metabolic rate (RMR)—the number of calories required for basic bodily processes such as tissue repair, brain function, blood circulation, digestion, and so on—plus the number of calories burned during exercise and normal daily activity.

Step 1: Determine Your Resting Metabolic Rate (RMR)

Women should use the following formula to determine their RMR:

$$655 + (\text{weight in kilograms} \times 9.6) +$$
$$(\text{height in centimeters} \times 1.8) - (\text{age} \times 4.7)$$

To convert pounds to kilograms, divide them by 2.2. To convert inches to centimeters, multiply them by 2.5. For example, if you are a forty-year-old woman who weighs 125 pounds and is 5 feet 6 inches tall, you would divide 125 by 2.2 to get 56.8 kilograms. Then you would multiply 66 inches by 2.5 to get a height of 165 centimeters. You would then get out your calculator and plug those figures into the equation to get your RMR.

$$\text{Weight: 56.8 kilograms} \times 9.6 = 545.28$$
$$\text{Height: 165 centimeters} \times 1.8 = 297$$
$$\text{Age: 40 years old} \times 4.7 = 188$$
$$\text{Finally: } (655 + 545.28 + 297) - 188 = 1,309 \text{ calories (RMR)}$$

Men should use this formula to compute their RMR:

$$66 + (\text{weight in kilograms} \times 13.7) +$$
$$(\text{height in centimeters} \times 5) - (\text{age} \times 6.8)$$

Since these formulas factor in gender, weight, height, and age, they are very precise and should be your preferred method for determining your RMR. However, a simple way to approximate your RMR is to multiply your body weight by 10. Using this formula, a 125-pound woman has a resting metabolic rate of 1,250 calories.

Step 2: Calculate the Caloric Value of Your Daily Activities

Since you don't sit around all day without moving a muscle, you need to account for the calories burned during exercise and physical activity. A good rule of thumb is that a person will burn about two-thirds of his or her body weight in calories for every 10 minutes of moderate cardiovascular exercise. So, a 125-pound woman would burn approximately 83.3 calories during every 10 minutes of her cardio workout.

To calculate the actual number of calories you will need to support your daily level of activity, use the following criteria:

- If you are very active throughout the day, add about 40–60 percent of your resting metabolic rate.
- If your daily activities are sedentary—for example, if you sit at a desk most of the day—add only 20 percent of your resting metabolic rate.

Let's look once again at our example of the 125-pound woman. If her RMR is 1,309 calories and she has a desk job, she would need to eat 1,309 + 261.8 = 1,570.8 calories daily to maintain her current weight. If she was moderately active, working out in the gym twice a week and doing aerobic exercises such as walking or bicycling five to six times per week, she would need to eat 1,309 + 523.6 = 1,832.6 calories daily to maintain her current weight.

Keep in mind that these numbers are only an estimate. Several factors can affect metabolic rate including age, genetics, certain medications, and body composition. Muscle is more metabolically active (burns more calories) than fat.

If you simply want to maintain your current weight, then you need to consume the number of calories you have determined as your total daily expenditure. If your goal is to lose weight, however, you'll need to cut back on your intake.

One pound of fat is equal to 3,500 calories. So, if you create a deficit of 500 calories a day, you should lose one pound each week. Take care not to slash too many calories, however, because you don't want to deprive your body of the nutrients it needs. Consuming fewer than 1,200 calories per day is not recommended.

Meal Plans for the 1,200-Calorie Program

The meal plans below, divided into options for breakfast, lunch, dinner, and snacks, are designed so that if you eat three meals per day and two snacks, you will be ingesting 1,200 calories. Each daily food plan includes 120 grams of carbohydrates, 90 grams of protein, and 40 grams of fat. Unless stated otherwise, one serving-size amount is assumed for foods from chapter 10.

Breakfast Options

½ cup cooked oatmeal with 1 Tbsp. ground flaxseed (optional); see Flavor-Bursting Oatmeal recipe for flavoring tips or stir 20 g whey protein powder into oatmeal.

2 low-fat and/or vegetarian sausage patties; try Healthy Choice, Morningstar Farms, or Boca varieties.

1 cup skim or soy milk, or 1 carton light yogurt (80–90 calories).

1 carton Egg Beaters, scrambled, with 1 thin slice each of cheddar cheese and lean ham, rolled into a small whole-wheat tortilla (look for at least 3 g fiber; we like La Tortilla Factory, with 8–9 g fiber per tortilla).

1 cup skim or soy milk, or 1 carton light yogurt (80–90 calories).

1 Eye-Opening Breakfast Burrito, using small (1 oz.) whole-wheat tortillas (see recipes).

1 cup skim or soy milk, or add 1 oz. cheese to burrito.

Vegetarian Frittata, using 4 egg whites only (see recipes), with ½ whole-wheat English muffin, toasted.

1 cup skim or soy milk.

1 slice 100% whole-grain bread (at least 3 g fiber per slice).

1 whole egg plus 2 egg whites, prepared any way you like (scrambled, over easy, etc.).

1 cup skim or soy milk, or add 1 oz. cheese to eggs.

1 whole-grain waffle (such as Kashi or Van's 7-grain frozen waffles), or made from a whole-wheat baking mix (such as Hodgeson Mills); top with 1 Tbsp. peanut butter (preferably natural peanut butter).

1 cup skim or soy milk.

½ cup whole-wheat pasta drizzled with 1 tsp. of olive oil (yes, it can be a great breakfast, for all you pasta lovers!); 2 oz. lean protein tossed in, such as chicken or shrimp.

Grab-and-Go fold-over sandwich with a glass of milk: 1 slice whole-grain bread, 2 slices turkey, and 1 thin slice cheese. Throw it together, fold it over, and you've got a great breakfast for the road.

Protein shake with 20 g whey protein (should contain no more than about 4 g carbohydrates per 20 g), 1 cup skim or soy milk, 1–2 Tbsp. ground flaxseed, and fresh or frozen berries (no sugar added). Add ice and blend.

Snack Options

Any time you are going more than four hours between meals, you should make sure you have a snack to keep your metabolism hot and your insulin levels even. Below are some suggestions for midmorning and midafternoon snacks.

1 small red apple with 1 Tbsp. almond butter.

5 whole-grain crackers (i.e., woven wheat crackers) topped with sliced mozzarella (approximately 1 oz.).

Trail Mix: 2 Tbsp. raisins with ½ oz. mixed nuts (approximately 10–12 nuts).

½ cup low-fat cottage cheese with 1 cup fresh berries.

Beef jerky (approximately 1 oz.) with 5 whole-grain crackers.

10–12 low-fat chips (i.e., Sun Chips, which have good fiber) with 3 Tbsp. bean dip or hummus.

1 whole-wheat tortilla topped with 3 Tbsp. shredded cheddar, melted. Roll up and dip into salsa.

1 small green apple, thinly sliced, tossed with ¼ avocado (cubed) and a splash of pear-infused vinegar (available at specialty and health food stores).

At smoothie store or a gym smoothie bar: Myoplex Lite blended with water is always a safe bet. Mackie's personal favorite flavor: Cappuccino Ice.

Protein Shake: Mix 20 g whey protein powder (should contain no more than about 4 g carbohydrates per 20 g) with 4 oz. water and 4 oz. skim or soy milk. Stir in 1 Tbsp. ground flaxseed (optional). Add ice and blend.

1 square dark chocolate (look for at least 70% cocoa) with 1 Tbsp. natural peanut butter.

Lunch Options

3 oz. seared tuna on a large bed of mixed greens, topped with 1 Tbsp. chopped walnuts and ½ cup whole-wheat croutons, drizzled with red wine vinaigrette to taste.

Orient Express Salad (see recipes).

Tuna, chicken, or salmon salad: Mix a 3-oz. can with ½ Tbsp. mayonnaise, pepper, and a splash of lemon juice. Serve over a bed of romaine with 5 whole-grain crackers.

3-oz. skinless chicken breast brushed lightly with barbecue sauce.
Spicy Roasted Sweet Potatoes (see recipes).
1–2 cups green beans sautéed with garlic.

½ cup whole-wheat pasta topped with ½ cup red sauce and 3 oz. ground turkey breast.
Spinach salad drizzled with 1–2 Tbsp. light Italian dressing.

Cabbage and Red Bean Soup (see recipes).
3 oz. grilled center-cut pork chop.

Southwestern Fajita (see recipes; use small whole-wheat tortilla and omit rice).

Greek Turkey Burger (see recipes) served on a lower-calorie wheat bun (approximately 80 calories per bun).

3 oz. grilled fish with ½ cup lentils and 1 medium broiled tomato.

3 oz. shrimp or crawfish stir-fried with mushrooms, spinach, onions, and minced garlic in 1 tsp. olive oil and a splash of soy sauce. Serve over ½ cup brown rice.

Whole-wheat tortilla wrap (we prefer La Tortilla Factory) with 2 oz. turkey, chicken, or lean ham, plus 1 thin slice cheese. Serve with Broccoli Medley (see recipes).

Pita Pocket Sandwich: Stuff 3 oz. of your favorite lean protein (turkey, chicken, tuna, lean roast beef or ham) into ½ whole-wheat pita (one pocket). Add fresh spinach leaves, sliced red peppers, and a drizzle of light vinaigrette dressing to taste.

Protein shake with 20 g whey protein (should contain no more than 4 g carbohydrates per 20 g), 1 cup skim or soy milk, 1–2 Tbsp. ground flaxseed, and ½ cup fresh or frozen berries (no sugar added). Add ice and blend.

Dinner Options

Key West Scallop Skewers (with 4 oz. scallops) with Spicy Sautéed Kale (see recipes).
Mixed greens salad with a splash of red wine vinaigrette to taste.

4 oz. grilled tuna or salmon.
1 large portobello mushroom and 1 sliced red pepper, grilled or roasted with 1 tsp. olive oil and seasonings.

Mexican-Style Lettuce Wraps (see recipes).

Shrimp Veggie Stir-Fry (see recipes).

Meatloaf (about ½ standard portion) with a serving of Grandma's Green Bean Pie (see recipes).

Chicken and Artichokes (see recipes).
Mixed green salad tossed with 1 Tbsp. light vinaigrette dressing.

Nirvana Kabobs with Baked Eggplant (see recipes).

Turkey Cutlets (see recipes).
1–2 cups steamed broccoli with 1–2 Tbsp. Parmesan cheese.

4 oz. pork tenderloin medallions.
Cauliflower "Potato Salad" (see recipes).
1–2 cups asparagus, steamed with a splash of lemon juice and a splash of balsamic vinegar.

Protein shake with 20 g whey protein (should contain no more than 4 g carbohydrates per 20 g), 1 cup skim or soy milk, 1–2 Tbsp. ground flaxseed, and ½ cup fresh or frozen berries (no sugar added). Add ice and blend.

Meal Plans for the 1,350-Calorie Program

The meal plans below, divided into options for breakfast, lunch, dinner, and snacks, are designed so that if you eat three meals per day and two snacks, you will be ingesting 1,350 calories. Each daily food plan includes

135 grams of carbohydrates, 100 grams of protein, and 45 grams of fat. Unless stated otherwise, one serving-size amount is assumed for foods from chapter 10.

Breakfast Options

1 cup cooked oatmeal with 1 Tbsp. ground flaxseed (optional); see Flavor-Bursting Oatmeal recipe for flavoring tips or stir 20 g whey protein powder into oatmeal.

2 low-fat and/or vegetarian sausage patties; try Healthy Choice, Morningstar Farms, or Boca varieties.

1 cup skim or soy milk, or 1 carton light yogurt.

1 carton Egg Beaters, scrambled, with 1 thin slice each of cheddar cheese and lean ham, rolled into a small whole-wheat tortilla (look for at least 3 g fiber; we like La Tortilla Factory, with 8–9 g fiber per tortilla).

2 small or 1 large kiwifruit.

1 cup skim or soy milk, or 1 carton light yogurt.

1 Eye-Opening Breakfast Burrito, using small (1 oz.) whole-wheat tortillas (see recipes). Add ⅓ cup canned black beans.

1 cup skim or soy milk, or add 1 oz. cheese to burrito.

Vegetarian Frittata, using 4 egg whites only (see recipes), with 1 whole-wheat English muffin, toasted.

1 medium green or red apple.

1 cup skim or soy milk.

2 slices 100% whole-grain bread (at least 3 g fiber per slice).

1 whole egg plus 2 egg whites, prepared any way you like (scrambled, over easy, etc.).

1 cup skim or soy milk, or add 1 oz. cheese to eggs.

1 whole-grain waffle (such as Kashi or Van's 7-grain frozen waffles), or made from a whole-wheat baking mix (such as Hodgeson Mills); top with 1 Tbsp. peanut butter (preferably natural peanut butter).

1 cup sliced strawberries.

1 cup skim or soy milk.

1 cup whole-wheat pasta drizzled with 1 tsp. olive oil (yes, it can be a great breakfast, for all you pasta lovers!); 2 oz. of lean protein tossed in, such as chicken or shrimp.

Grab-and-Go sandwich with a glass of milk: 2 slices whole-grain bread, 2 slices turkey, and 1 thin slice cheese. Throw it together, and you've got a great breakfast for the road.

Protein shake with 20 g whey protein (should contain no more than about 4 g carbohydrates per 20 g), 1 cup skim or soy milk, 1–2 Tbsp. ground flaxseed, and ½ cup fresh or frozen berries (no sugar added). Add ice and blend.
1 slice whole-grain bread, or 1 serving (4 oz.) fresh fruit.

Snack Options

Any time you are going more than four hours between meals, you should make sure you have a snack to keep your metabolism hot and your insulin levels even. Below are some suggestions for midmorning and midafternoon snacks.

1 small red apple with 1 Tbsp. almond butter.

5 whole-grain crackers (i.e., woven wheat crackers) topped with sliced mozzarella (approximately 1 oz.).

Trail Mix: 2 Tbsp. raisins with ½ oz. mixed nuts (approximately 10–12 nuts).

½ cup low-fat cottage cheese with 1 cup fresh berries.

Beef jerky (approximately 1 oz.) with 5 whole-grain crackers.

10–12 low-fat chips (i.e., Sun Chips, which have good fiber) with 3 Tbsp. bean dip or hummus.

1 whole-wheat tortilla topped with 3 Tbsp. shredded cheddar, melted. Roll up and dip into salsa.

1 small green apple, thinly sliced, tossed with ½ avocado (cubed) and a splash of pear-infused vinegar (available at specialty and health food stores).

At smoothie store or a gym smoothie bar: Myoplex Lite blended with water is always a safe bet. Mackie's personal favorite flavor: Cappuccino Ice.

Protein Shake: Mix 20 g whey protein powder (should contain no more than about 4 g carbohydrates per 20 g) with 4 oz. water and 4 oz. skim or soy milk. Stir in 1 Tbsp. ground flaxseed (optional). Add ice and blend.

1 square dark chocolate (look for at least 70% cocoa) with 1 Tbsp. natural peanut butter.

Lunch Options

4 oz. seared tuna on a large bed of mixed greens, topped with 1 Tbsp. chopped walnuts and ½ cup whole-wheat croutons, drizzled with red wine vinaigrette.

Orient Express Salad (see recipes). Add 1 Tbsp. slivered almonds.

Tuna, chicken, or salmon salad: Mix 4 oz. with ½ Tbsp. mayonnaise, pepper, and a splash of lemon juice. Serve over a bed of romaine with 5 whole-grain crackers.

4-oz. skinless chicken breast brushed lightly with barbecue sauce.
Spicy Roasted Sweet Potatoes (see recipes).
1–2 cups green beans sautéed with garlic.

½ cup whole-wheat pasta topped with ½ cup red sauce and 4 oz. ground turkey breast.
Spinach salad drizzled with 1–2 Tbsp. light Italian dressing.

Cabbage and Red Bean Soup (see recipes).
4 oz. grilled center-cut pork chop.

Southwestern Fajita (see recipes; use small whole-wheat tortilla, and omit rice).

Greek Turkey Burger (see recipes) served on a lower-calorie wheat bun (approximately 80 calories per bun). Add ½ oz. of your favorite cheese, thinly sliced.

4 oz. grilled fish with ½ cup lentils and 1 medium broiled tomato.

4 oz. shrimp or crawfish stir-fried with mushrooms, spinach, onions, and minced garlic in 1 tsp. olive oil and a splash of soy sauce. Serve over ⅓ cup brown rice.

Whole-wheat tortilla wrap (we prefer La Tortilla Factory) with 3 oz. turkey, chicken, or lean ham, plus 1 thin slice cheese. Serve with Broccoli Medley (see recipes).

Pita Pocket Sandwich: Stuff 4 oz. of your favorite lean protein (turkey, chicken, tuna, lean roast beef or ham) into ½ whole-wheat pita (one pocket). Add fresh spinach leaves, sliced red peppers, and a drizzle of light vinaigrette dressing to taste.

Protein shake with 25 g whey protein (should contain no more than 4 g carbohydrates per 20 g), 1 cup skim or soy milk, 1–2 Tbsp. ground flaxseed, and ½ cup fresh or frozen berries (no sugar added). Add ice and blend.

Dinner Options

Key West Scallop Skewers (with 4 oz. scallops) with Spicy Sautéed Kale (see recipes).
Mixed greens salad with a splash of red wine vinaigrette to taste.

4 oz. grilled tuna or salmon.
1 large portobello mushroom and 1 sliced red pepper, grilled or roasted with 1 tsp. olive oil and seasonings.

Mexican-Style Lettuce Wraps (see recipes).

Shrimp Veggie Stir-Fry (see recipes).

Meatloaf (about ½ standard portion) with a serving of Grandma's Green Bean Pie (see recipes).

Chicken and Artichokes (see recipes).
Mixed green salad tossed with 1 Tbsp. light vinaigrette dressing.

Nirvana Kabobs with Baked Eggplant (see recipes).

Turkey Cutlets (see recipes).
1–2 cups steamed broccoli with 1–2 Tbsp. Parmesan cheese.

4 oz. pork tenderloin medallions.
Cauliflower "Potato Salad" (see recipes).
1–2 cups asparagus, steamed with a splash of lemon juice and a splash of balsamic vinegar.

Protein shake with 20 g whey protein (should contain no more than 4 g carbohydrates per 20 g), 1 cup skim or soy milk, 1–2 Tbsp. ground flaxseed, and ½ cup fresh or frozen berries (no sugar added). Add ice and blend.

Meal Plans for the 1,500-Calorie Program

The meal plans below, divided into options for breakfast, lunch, dinner, and snacks, are designed so that if you eat three meals per day and two snacks, you will be ingesting 1,500 calories. Each daily food plan includes 150 grams of carbohydrates, 112 grams of protein, 50 grams of fat. Unless stated otherwise, one serving-size amount is assumed for foods from chapter 10.

Breakfast Options

1 cup cooked oatmeal with 1 Tbsp. ground flaxseed (optional); see Flavor-Bursting Oatmeal recipe for flavoring tips or stir 20 g whey protein powder into oatmeal.

2 low-fat and/or vegetarian sausage patties; try Healthy Choice, Morningstar Farms, or Boca varieties.

1 cup skim or soy milk, or 1 carton light yogurt.

1 carton Egg Beaters, scrambled, with 1 thin slice each of cheddar cheese and lean ham, rolled into a small whole-wheat tortilla (look for at least 3 g fiber; we like La Tortilla Factory, with 8–9 g fiber per tortilla).

2 small or 1 large kiwi fruit.

1 cup skim or soy milk, or 1 carton light yogurt.

1 Eye-Opening Breakfast Burrito, using small (1 oz.) whole-wheat tortillas (see recipes). Add ⅓ cup canned black beans.

1 cup skim or soy milk, or add 1 oz. cheese to burrito.

Vegetarian Frittata, with 4 egg whites only (see recipes), with 1 whole-wheat English muffin, toasted.

1 medium green or red apple.

1 cup skim or soy milk.

2 slices 100% whole-grain bread (at least 3 g fiber per slice).

1 whole egg plus 2 egg whites, prepared any way you like (scrambled, over easy, etc.).

1 cup skim or soy milk, or add 1 oz. cheese to eggs.

1 whole-grain waffle (such as Kashi or Van's 7-grain frozen waffles), or made from a whole-wheat baking mix (such as Hodgeson Mills); top with 1 Tbsp. peanut butter (preferably natural peanut butter).

1 cup sliced strawberries.

1 cup skim or soy milk.

1 cup whole-wheat pasta drizzled with 1 tsp. olive oil (yes, it can be a great breakfast, for all you pasta lovers!); 2 oz. lean protein tossed in, such as chicken or shrimp.

Grab-and-Go sandwich with a glass of milk: 2 slices whole-grain bread, 2 slices turkey, and 1 thin slice cheese. Throw it together, and you've got a great breakfast for the road.

Protein shake with 20 g whey protein (should contain no more than 4 g carbohydrates per 20 g), 1 cup skim or soy milk, 1–2 Tbsp. ground flaxseed, and ½ cup fresh or frozen berries (no sugar added). Add ice and blend.
1 slice whole-grain bread, or ½ cup fresh fruit.

Snack Options

Any time you are going more than four hours between meals, you should make sure you have a snack to keep your metabolism hot and your insulin levels even. Below are some suggestions for midmorning and midafternoon snacks.

1 small red apple with 1 Tbsp. almond butter.

5 whole-grain crackers (i.e., woven wheat crackers) topped with sliced mozzarella (approximately 1 oz.).

Trail Mix: 2 Tbsp. raisins with ½ oz. mixed nuts (approximately 10–12 nuts).

½ cup low-fat cottage cheese with 1 cup fresh berries.

Beef jerky (approximately 1 oz.) with 5 whole-grain crackers.

10–12 low-fat chips (i.e., Sun Chips, which have good fiber) with 3 Tbsp. bean dip or hummus.

1 whole-wheat tortilla topped with 3 Tbsp. shredded cheddar, melted. Roll up and dip into salsa.

1 small green apple, thinly sliced, tossed with ¼ avocado (cubed) and a splash of pear-infused vinegar (available at specialty and health food stores).

At smoothie store or a gym smoothie bar: Myoplex Lite blended with water is always a safe bet. Mackie's personal favorite flavor: Cappuccino Ice.

Protein Shake: Mix 20 g whey protein powder (should contain no more than 4 grams carbohydrates per 20 g) with 4 oz. water and 4 oz. skim or soy milk. Stir in 1 Tbsp. ground flaxseed (optional). Add ice and blend.

1 square dark chocolate (look for at least 70% cocoa) with 1 Tbsp. natural peanut butter.

Lunch Options

4 oz. seared tuna on a large bed of mixed greens, topped with 1 Tbsp. chopped walnuts and ½ cup whole-wheat croutons, drizzled with red wine vinaigrette.

Orient Express Salad (see recipes). Add 1 Tbsp. slivered almonds.

Tuna, chicken, or salmon salad: Mix 4 oz. with ½ Tbsp. mayonnaise, pepper, and a splash of lemon juice. Serve over a bed of romaine with 5 whole-grain crackers.

4-oz. skinless chicken breast brushed lightly with barbecue sauce.
Spicy Roasted Sweet Potatoes (see recipes).
1–2 cups green beans sautéed with garlic.

½ cup whole-wheat pasta topped with ½ cup red sauce and 4 oz. ground turkey breast.
Spinach salad drizzled with 1–2 Tbsp. light Italian dressing.

Cabbage and Red Bean Soup (see recipes).
4 oz. grilled center-cut pork chop.

Southwestern Fajita (see recipes; use small whole-wheat tortilla, and omit rice).

Greek Turkey Burger (see recipes) served on a lower-calorie wheat bun (approximately 80 calories per bun). Add your favorite cheese, 2 oz. thinly sliced.

4 oz. grilled fish with ½ cup lentils and 1 medium broiled tomato.

4 oz. shrimp or crawfish stir-fried with mushrooms, spinach, onions, and minced garlic in 1 tsp. olive oil and a splash of soy sauce. Serve over ⅓ cup brown rice.

Whole-wheat tortilla wrap (we prefer La Tortilla Factory) with 3 oz. turkey, chicken, or lean ham, plus 1 thin slice cheese. Serve with Broccoli Medley (see recipes).

Pita Pocket Sandwich: Stuff 4 oz. of your favorite lean protein (turkey, chicken, tuna, lean roast beef or ham) into ½ whole-wheat pita (one pocket). Add fresh spinach leaves, sliced red peppers, and a drizzle of light vinaigrette dressing to taste.

Protein shake with 25 g whey protein (should contain no more than 4 g carbohydrates per 20 g), 1 cup skim or soy milk, 1–2 Tbsp. ground flaxseed, and ½ cup fresh or frozen berries (no sugar added). Add ice and blend.

Dinner Options

Key West Scallop Skewers (with 5–6 oz. scallops) with Spicy Sautéed Kale (see recipes).
Mixed greens salad with a splash of red wine vinaigrette to taste.
½ cup Zesty Black Beans, without rice (see recipes).

5 oz. grilled tuna or salmon.
1 large portobello mushroom and 1 sliced red pepper, grilled or roasted with 1 tsp. olive oil and seasonings.
½ cup couscous.

Mexican-Style Lettuce Wraps, using 5 oz. chicken, 1 small whole-wheat tortilla for one wrap and lettuce for rest (see recipes).

Shrimp Veggie Stir-Fry, using 5–6 oz. shrimp (see recipes). Serve over ½ cup basmati rice.

Mushroom and Spinach Pizza (see recipes). Add 3 oz. shrimp, turkey pepperoni, or diced chicken.

Meatloaf with a serving of Grandma's Green Bean Pie (see recipes).
3 oz. baked sweet potato flavored to taste with cinnamon and vanilla extract.

Chicken and Artichokes (see recipes).
½ cup whole-wheat penne pasta with 1–2 Tbsp. olive oil and 1–2 Tbsp. Parmesan.
Mixed green salad tossed with 1 Tbsp. light vinaigrette dressing.

Nirvana Kabobs with Baked Eggplant (see recipes).
½ cup Flax-Fortified Fried Rice without sirloin (see recipes).

5 oz. pork tenderloin medallions.
Cauliflower "Potato Salad" (see recipes).
1–2 cups asparagus, steamed with a splash of lemon juice and a splash of balsamic vinegar.
1 whole-wheat dinner roll.

Protein shake with 20 g whey protein (should contain no more than 4 g carbohydrates per 20 g), 1 cup skim or soy milk, 1–2 Tbsp. ground flaxseed, and ½ cup fresh or frozen berries (no sugar added). Add ice and blend.

5–8 whole-grain crackers with 1 thin slice cheese.

Meal Plans for the 1,600-Calorie Program

The meal plans below, divided into options for breakfast, lunch, dinner, and snacks, are designed so that if you eat three meals per day and three snacks, you will be ingesting 1,600 calories. Each daily food plan includes 160 grams of carbohydrates, 120 grams of protein, and 53 grams of fat. Unless stated otherwise, one serving-size amount is assumed for foods from chapter 10.

Breakfast Options

1 cup cooked oatmeal with 1 Tbsp. ground flaxseed (optional); see Flavor-Bursting Oatmeal recipe for flavoring tips or stir 20 g whey protein powder into oatmeal.

2 low-fat and/or vegetarian sausage patties; try Healthy Choice, Morningstar Farms, or Boca varieties.

1 cup skim or soy milk, or 1 carton light yogurt.

1 carton Egg Beaters, scrambled, with 1 thin slice each of cheddar cheese and lean ham, rolled into a small whole-wheat tortilla (look for at least 3 g fiber; we like La Tortilla Factory, with 8–9 g fiber per tortilla).

2 small or 1 large kiwifruit.

1 cup skim or soy milk, or 1 carton light yogurt.

1 Eye-Opening Breakfast Burrito, using small (1 oz.) whole-wheat tortillas (see recipes). Add ⅓ cup canned black beans.

1 cup skim or soy milk, or add 1 oz. cheese to burrito.

Vegetarian Frittata, with 4 egg whites only (see recipes), with 1 whole-wheat English muffin, toasted.

1 medium green or red apple.

1 cup skim or soy milk.

2 slices 100% whole-grain bread (at least 3 g fiber per slice).

1 whole egg plus 2 egg whites, prepared any way you like (scrambled, over easy, etc.).

1 cup skim or soy milk, or add 1 oz. cheese to eggs.

1 whole-grain waffle (such as Kashi or Van's 7-grain frozen waffles), or made from a whole-wheat baking mix (such as Hodgeson Mills); top with 1 Tbsp. peanut butter (preferably natural peanut butter).

1 cup sliced strawberries.

1 cup skim or soy milk.

1 cup whole-wheat pasta drizzled with 1 tsp. olive oil (yes, it can be a great breakfast, for all you pasta lovers!); 2 oz. lean protein tossed in, such as chicken or shrimp.

Grab-and-Go sandwich with a glass of milk: 2 slices whole-grain bread, 2 slices turkey, and 1 thin slice cheese. Throw it together, and you've got a great breakfast for the road.

Protein shake with 20 g whey protein (should contain no more than 4 g carbohydrates per 20 g), 1 cup skim or soy milk, 1–2 Tbsp. ground flaxseed, and ½ cup fresh or frozen berries (no sugar added). Add ice and blend.

1 slice whole-grain bread, or ½ cup fresh fruit.

Snack Options

Any time you are going more than four hours between meals, you should make sure you have a snack to keep your metabolism hot and your insulin levels even. Below are some suggestions for midmorning, midafternoon, and before-bedtime snacks.

1 small red apple with 1½ Tbsp. almond butter.

5 whole-grain crackers (i.e., woven wheat crackers) topped with sliced mozzarella (approximately 1½ oz.).

Trail Mix: 2 Tbsp. raisins with 1 oz. mixed nuts (approximately ¼ cup).

1 cup low-fat cottage cheese with 1 cup fresh berries.

Beef jerky (approximately 2 oz.) with 5 whole-grain crackers.

15–16 low-fat chips (i.e., Sun Chips, which have good fiber) with ¼ cup bean dip or hummus.

1 whole-wheat tortilla topped with ¼ cup shredded cheddar, melted. Roll up and dip into salsa and 1 Tbsp. light sour cream.

1 large green apple, thinly sliced, tossed with ¼ avocado (cubed) and a splash of pear-infused vinegar (available at specialty and health food stores).

At smoothie store or a gym smoothie bar: Myoplex Lite blended with water and berries is always a safe bet. Mackie's personal favorite flavor: Cappuccino Ice.

Protein Shake: Mix 20 g whey protein powder (should contain no more than 4 g carbohydrates per 20 g) with 1 cup skim or soy milk. Stir in 1 Tbsp. ground flaxseed (optional). Add ice and blend.

1 square dark chocolate (look for at least 70% cocoa) with 1½ Tbsp. natural peanut butter.

Lunch Options

4 oz. seared tuna on a large bed of mixed greens, topped with 1 Tbsp. chopped walnuts and ½ cup whole-wheat croutons, drizzled with red wine vinaigrette.

Orient Express Salad (see recipes). Add 1 Tbsp. slivered almonds.

Tuna, chicken, or salmon salad: Mix 4 oz. with ½ Tbsp. mayonnaise, pepper, and a splash of lemon juice. Serve over a bed of romaine with 5 whole-grain crackers.

4-oz. skinless chicken breast brushed lightly with barbecue sauce.
Spicy Roasted Sweet Potatoes (see recipes).
1–2 cups green beans sautéed with garlic.

½ cup whole-wheat pasta topped with ½ cup red sauce and 4 oz. ground turkey breast.
Spinach salad drizzled with 1–2 Tbsp. light Italian dressing.

Cabbage and Red Bean Soup (see recipes).
4 oz. grilled center-cut pork chop.

Southwestern Fajita (see recipes; use small whole-wheat tortilla, and omit rice).

Greek Turkey Burger (see recipes) served on a lower-calorie wheat bun (approximately 80 calories per bun). Add your favorite cheese, 2 oz. thinly sliced.

4 oz. grilled fish with ½ cup lentils and 1 medium broiled tomato.

4 oz. shrimp or crawfish stir-fried with mushrooms, spinach, onions, and minced garlic in 1 tsp. olive oil and a splash of soy sauce. Serve over ⅓ cup brown rice.

Whole-wheat tortilla wrap (we prefer La Tortilla Factory) with 3 oz. turkey, chicken, or lean ham, plus 1 thin slice cheese. Serve with Broccoli Medley (see recipes).

Pita Pocket Sandwich: Stuff 4 oz. of your favorite lean protein (turkey, chicken, tuna, lean roast beef or ham) into ½ whole-wheat pita (one pocket). Add fresh spinach leaves, sliced red peppers, and 1–2 Tbsp. light vinaigrette dressing.

Protein shake with 25 g whey protein (should contain no more than 4 g carbohydrates per 20 g), 1 cup skim or soy milk, 1–2 Tbsp. ground flaxseed, and ½ cup fresh or frozen berries (no sugar added). Add ice and blend.

Dinner Options

Key West Scallop Skewers (with 5–6 oz. scallops) with Spicy Sautéed Kale (see recipes).
Mixed greens salad with a splash of red wine vinaigrette to taste.
½ cup Zesty Black Beans, without rice (see recipes).

5 oz. grilled tuna or salmon.
Portobello mushrooms and red peppers, grilled or roasted with 1 tsp. olive oil and seasonings.
½ cup couscous.

Mexican-Style Lettuce Wraps, using 5 oz. chicken, 1 small whole-wheat tortilla for one wrap and lettuce for rest (see recipes).

Shrimp Veggie Stir-Fry, using 5–6 oz. shrimp (see recipes). Serve over ½ cup basmati rice.

Mushroom and Spinach Pizza (see recipes). Add 4 oz. shrimp, turkey pepperoni, or diced chicken.

Meatloaf with a serving of Grandma's Green Bean Pie (see recipes).
3 oz. baked sweet potato flavored with cinnamon and vanilla extract to taste.

Chicken and Artichokes (see recipes).
½ cup whole-wheat penne pasta with a drizzle of olive oil and 1–2 Tbsp. Parmesan.
Mixed green salad tossed with 1 Tbsp. light vinaigrette dressing.

Nirvana Kabobs with Baked Eggplant (see recipes).
½ cup Flax-Fortified Fried Rice without sirloin (see recipes).

5 oz. pork tenderloin medallions.

Cauliflower "Potato Salad" (see recipes).

1–2 cups asparagus, steamed with a splash of lemon juice and a splash of balsamic vinegar.

1 whole-wheat dinner roll.

Protein shake with 20 g whey protein (should contain no more than 4 g carbohydrates per 20 g), 1 cup skim or soy milk, 1–2 Tbsp. ground flaxseed, and ½ cup fresh or frozen berries (no sugar added). Add ice and blend.

5–8 whole grain-crackers with 1 thin slice cheese.

Nighttime Snack Options

1 cup skim or soy milk; add a splash of vanilla or almond extract to flavor it.

1 carton light yogurt.

½ cup no sugar-added ice cream (we like Blue Bell Light).

½ cup low-fat cottage cheese; add 1 Tbsp. light yogurt or a little Splenda to flavor it.

1 cup sugar-free pudding made with skim milk.

1 oz. cheese, any variety.

Meal Plans for the 1,800-Calorie Program

The meal plans below, divided into options for breakfast, lunch, dinner, and snacks, are designed so that if you eat three meals per day and three snacks, you will be ingesting 1,800 calories. Each daily food plan includes 180 grams of carbohydrates, 135 grams of protein, 60 grams of fat. Unless stated otherwise, one serving-size amount is assumed for foods from chapter 10.

Breakfast Options

1 cup cooked oatmeal with 1 Tbsp. ground flaxseed (optional); see Flavor-Bursting Oatmeal recipe for flavoring tips or stir 20 g whey protein powder into oatmeal.

2 low-fat and/or vegetarian sausage patties; try Healthy Choice, Morningstar Farms, or Boca varieties.

1 cup skim or soy milk, or 1 carton light yogurt.

1 small carton Egg Beaters, scrambled, with 1 thin slice each of cheddar cheese and lean ham, rolled into a small whole-wheat tortilla (look for at least 3 g fiber; we like La Tortilla Factory, with 8–9 g of fiber per tortilla).

2 small or 1 large kiwifruit.

1 cup skim or soy milk, or 1 carton light yogurt.

1 Eye-Opening Breakfast Burrito, using small (1 oz.) whole-wheat tortillas (see recipes). Add ⅓ cup canned black beans.

1 cup skim or soy milk, or add 1 oz. cheese to burrito.

Vegetarian Frittata, with egg whites only (see recipes), with 1 whole-wheat English muffin, toasted.

1 medium green or red apple.

1 cup skim or soy milk.

2 slices 100% whole-grain bread (at least 3 g fiber per slice).

1 whole egg plus 2 egg whites, prepared any way you like (scrambled, over easy, etc.).

1 cup skim or soy milk, or add 1 oz. cheese to eggs.

1 whole-grain waffle (such as Kashi or Van's 7-grain frozen waffles), or made from a whole-wheat baking mix (such as Hodgeson Mills); top with 1 Tbsp. peanut butter (preferably natural peanut butter).

1 cup sliced strawberries.

1 cup skim or soy milk.

1 cup whole-wheat pasta drizzled with 1 tsp. olive oil (yes, it can be a great breakfast, for all you pasta lovers!); 2 oz. lean protein tossed in, such as chicken or shrimp.

Grab-and-Go sandwich with a glass of milk: 2 slices whole-grain bread, 2 slices turkey, and 1 thin slice cheese. Throw it together, and you've got a great breakfast for the road.

Protein shake with 20 g whey protein (should contain no more than 4 g carbohydrates per 20 g), 1 cup skim or soy milk, 1–2 Tbsp. ground flaxseed, and ½ cup fresh or frozen berries (no sugar added). Add ice and blend.

1 slice whole-grain bread, or 4 oz. fresh fruit.

Snack Options

Any time you are going more than four hours between meals, you should make sure you have a snack to keep your metabolism hot and your insulin levels even. Below are some suggestions for midmorning, midafternoon, and before-bedtime snacks.

1 small red apple with 2 Tbsp. almond butter.

5 whole-grain crackers (i.e., woven wheat crackers) topped with sliced mozzarella (approximately 2 oz.).

Trail Mix: 2 Tbsp. raisins with 1 oz. mixed nuts (approximately 20–24 nuts).

1 cup low-fat cottage cheese topped with 1 cup fresh berries and 1 Tbsp. sunflower seeds.

Beef jerky (approximately 2 oz.) with 8 whole-grain crackers.

20 low-fat chips (i.e., Sun Chips, which have good fiber) with ¼ cup bean dip or hummus.

1 whole-wheat tortilla topped with ¼ cup diced skinless chicken breast and ¼ cup shredded cheddar, melted. Roll up and dip into salsa and 1 Tbsp. sour cream.

1 small green apple, thinly sliced, tossed with ½ avocado (cubed) and a splash of pear-infused vinegar (available in specialty and health food stores).

At smoothie store or a gym smoothie bar: Myoplex Lite blended with water and berries is always a safe bet. Mackie's personal favorite flavor: Cappuccino Ice.

Protein Shake: Mix 20 g whey protein powder (should contain no more than 4 g carbohydrates per 20 g), with 1 cup skim or soy milk and 1 cup berries (no sugar added). Stir in 1 Tbsp. ground flaxseed (optional). Add ice and blend.

1 square dark chocolate (look for at least 70% cocoa) with 2 Tbsp. natural peanut butter.

Lunch Options

4 oz. seared tuna on a large bed of mixed greens, topped with ½ mango, cubed, and 1 Tbsp. chopped walnuts, with ½ cup whole-wheat croutons, drizzled with red wine vinaigrette to taste.

Orient Express Salad (see recipes). Add 1 Tbsp. slivered almonds and ½ cup soybeans.

Tuna, chicken, or salmon salad: Mix 4 oz. with ½ Tbsp. mayonnaise, pepper, and a splash of lemon juice. Add ½ cup red grapes, halved. Serve over a bed of romaine with 5 whole-grain crackers.

4-oz. skinless chicken breast brushed lightly with barbecue sauce.
2 servings Spicy Roasted Sweet Potatoes (see recipes).
1–2 cups green beans sautéed with garlic.

1 cup whole-wheat pasta topped with ½ cup red sauce and 4 oz. ground turkey breast.
Spinach salad drizzled with 1–2 Tbsp. light Italian dressing.

Cabbage and Red Bean Soup served over ⅓ cup basmati rice (see recipes).
4 oz. grilled center-cut pork chop.

Southwestern Fajita (see recipes; use two small whole-wheat tortillas).

Greek Turkey Burger (see recipes) served on a lower-calorie wheat bun (approximately 80 calories per bun). Add your favorite cheese, 2 oz., thinly sliced.
3 oz. sweet potato flavored with cinnamon and Splenda (optional).

4 oz. grilled fish with 1 cup lentils and 1 medium broiled tomato.

4 oz. shrimp or crawfish stir-fried with mushrooms, spinach, onions, and minced garlic in 1 tsp. olive oil and a splash of soy sauce. Serve over ⅔ cup brown rice.

Whole-wheat tortilla wrap (we prefer La Tortilla Factory) with 3 oz. turkey, chicken, or lean ham, plus 1 thin slice cheese. Dip into 4 Tbsp. hummus (or spread hummus over tortilla before wrapping). Serve with Broccoli Medley (see recipes).

Pita Pocket Sandwich: Stuff 4 oz. of your favorite lean protein (turkey, chicken, tuna, lean roast beef or ham) into a whole-wheat pita (both pockets). Add fresh spinach leaves, sliced red peppers, and a drizzle of light vinaigrette dressing.

Protein shake with 25 g whey protein (should contain no more than 4 g carbohydrates per 20 g), 1 cup skim or soy milk, 1–2 Tbsp. ground flaxseed, and ½ cup fresh or frozen berries (no sugar added). Add ice and blend.
5 whole-grain crackers or a piece of fruit.

Dinner Options

Key West Scallop Skewers (with 5–6 oz. scallops) with Spicy Sautéed Kale (see recipes).

Mixed greens salad with a splash of red wine vinaigrette to taste.

½ cup Zesty Black Beans, without rice (see recipes).

5 oz. grilled tuna or salmon.

1 large portobello mushroom and 1 sliced red pepper, grilled or roasted with 1 tsp. olive oil and seasonings.

½ cup couscous.

Mexican-Style Lettuce Wraps, using 5 oz. chicken, 1 small whole-wheat tortilla for one wrap and lettuce for rest (see recipes).

Shrimp Veggie Stir-Fry, using 5–6 oz. shrimp (see recipes). Serve over ½ cup basmati rice.

Mushroom and Spinach Pizza (see recipes). Add 5 oz. shrimp, turkey pepperoni, or diced chicken.

Meatloaf with a serving of Grandma's Green Bean Pie (see recipes).

3 oz. baked sweet potato flavored with cinnamon and vanilla extract to taste.

Chicken and Artichokes (see recipes).

½ cup whole-wheat penne pasta with a drizzle of olive oil and 1 oz. Parmesan.

Mixed green salad tossed with 1 Tbsp. light vinaigrette dressing.

Nirvana Kabobs with Baked Eggplant (see recipes).

½ cup Flax-Fortified Fried Rice without sirloin (see recipes).

5 oz. pork tenderloin medallions.

Cauliflower "Potato Salad" (see recipes).

1–2 cups asparagus, steamed with a splash of lemon juice and a splash of balsamic vinegar.

1 whole-wheat dinner roll.

Protein shake with 30 g whey protein (should contain no more than 6 g carbohydrates per 30 g), 1 cup skim or soy milk, 1–2 Tbsp. ground flaxseed, and ½ cup fresh or frozen berries (no sugar added). Add ice and blend.

5–8 whole-grain crackers topped with 1 thin slice cheese.

Nighttime Snack Options

1 cup skim or soy milk; add a splash of vanilla or almond extract to flavor it.

1 carton light yogurt.

½ cup no-sugar-added ice cream (we like Blue Bell Light).

½ cup low-fat cottage cheese; add 1 Tbsp. of light yogurt or a little Splenda to flavor it.

1 cup sugar-free pudding made with skim milk.

1 oz. cheese, any variety.

Meal Plans for the 2,000-Calorie Program

The meal plans below, divided into options for breakfast, lunch, dinner, and snacks, are designed so that if you eat three meals per day and three snacks, you will be ingesting 2,000 calories. Each daily food plan includes 200 grams of carbohydrates, 150 grams of protein, and 66 grams of fat. Unless stated otherwise, one serving-size amount is assumed for foods from chapter 10.

Breakfast Options

1 cup cooked oatmeal with 1 Tbsp. ground flaxseed (optional); see Flavor-Bursting Oatmeal recipe for flavoring tips or stir 20 g whey protein powder into oatmeal.
2 low-fat and/or vegetarian sausage patties; try Healthy Choice, Morningstar Farms, or Boca varieties.
1 cup skim or soy milk, or 1 carton light yogurt.

1 carton Egg Beaters, scrambled, with 1 thin slice each of cheddar cheese and lean ham, rolled into a small whole-wheat tortilla (look for at least 3 g fiber; we like La Tortilla Factory, with 8–9 g fiber per tortilla).
2 small or 1 large kiwifruit.
1 cup skim or soy milk (or 1 carton light yogurt).

1 Eye-Opening Breakfast Burrito, using small (1-oz.) whole-wheat tortillas (see recipes). Add ⅓ cup canned black beans.
1 cup skim or soy milk, or add 1 oz. cheese to burrito.

Vegetarian Frittata, with 4 egg whites only (see recipes), with 1 whole-wheat
English muffin, toasted.

1 medium green or red apple.

1 cup skim or soy milk.

2 slices 100% whole-grain bread (at least 3 g fiber per slice).

1 whole egg plus 2 egg whites, prepared any way you like (scrambled, over easy,
etc.).

1 cup skim or soy milk, or add 1 oz. cheese to eggs.

1 whole-grain waffle (such as Kashi or Van's 7-grain frozen waffles), or made
from a whole-wheat baking mix (such as Hodgeson Mills); top with 1 Tbsp.
peanut butter (preferably natural peanut butter).

1 cup sliced strawberries.

1 cup skim or soy milk.

1 cup whole-wheat pasta drizzled with 1 tsp. olive oil (yes, it can be a great
breakfast, for all you pasta lovers!); 2 oz. lean protein tossed in, such as
chicken or shrimp.

Grab-and-Go sandwich with a glass of milk: 2 slices whole-grain bread, 2 slices
turkey, and 1 thin slice cheese. Throw it together, and you've got a great
breakfast for the road.

Protein shake with 20 g whey protein (should contain no more than 4 g
carbohydrates per 20 g), 1 cup skim or soy milk, 1–2 Tbsp. ground flaxseed,
and ½ cup fresh or frozen berries (no sugar added). Add ice and blend.

1 slice whole-grain bread, or 2 oz. fresh fruit.

Snack Options

Any time you are going more than four hours between meals, you should
make sure you have a snack to keep your metabolism hot and your insulin
levels even. Below are some suggestions for midmorning, midafternoon,
and before-bedtime snacks.

1 small red apple with 2 Tbsp. almond butter.

5 whole-grain crackers (i.e., woven wheat crackers) topped with sliced
mozzarella (approximately 2 oz.).

Trail Mix: 2 Tbsp. raisins with 1 oz. mixed nuts (approximately 20–24 nuts).

1 cup low-fat cottage cheese topped with 1 cup fresh berries and 1 Tbsp. sunflower seeds.

Beef jerky (approximately 2 oz.) with 8 whole-grain crackers.

20 low-fat chips (i.e., Sun Chips, which have good fiber) with ¼ cup bean dip or hummus.

1 whole-wheat tortilla topped with ¼ cup diced skinless chicken breast and ¼ cup shredded cheddar, melted. Roll up and dip into salsa and 1 Tbsp. sour cream.

1 small green apple, thinly sliced, tossed with ½ avocado (cubed) and a splash of pear-infused vinegar (available at specialty and health food stores).

At smoothie store or a gym smoothie bar: Myoplex Lite blended with water and berries is always a safe bet. Mackie's personal favorite flavor: Cappuccino Ice.

Protein Shake: Mix 20 g whey protein powder (should contain no more than 4 g carbohydrates per 20 g) with 1 cup skim or soy milk and 1 cup berries (no sugar added). Stir in 1 Tbsp. ground flaxseed (optional). Add ice and blend.

1 square dark chocolate (look for at least 70% cocoa) with 2 Tbsp. natural peanut butter.

Lunch Options

5 oz. seared tuna on a large bed of mixed greens, topped with ½ mango, cubed, and 1 Tbsp. chopped walnuts, with ½ cup whole-wheat croutons, drizzled with red wine vinaigrette to taste.

Orient Express Salad (see recipes). Add 2 oz. diced chicken breast, 1 Tbsp. slivered almonds, and ½ cup soybeans.

Tuna, chicken, or salmon salad: Mix 5 oz. with ½ Tbsp. mayonnaise, pepper, and a splash of lemon juice. Add ½ cup red grapes, halved. Serve over a bed of romaine with 5 whole-grain crackers.

5-oz. skinless chicken breast brushed lightly with barbecue sauce.
2 servings Spicy Roasted Sweet Potatoes (see recipes).
1–2 cups green beans sautéed with garlic.

1 cup whole-wheat pasta topped with ½ cup red sauce and 5 oz. ground turkey breast.

Spinach salad drizzled with 1–2 Tbsp. light Italian dressing.

Cabbage and Red Bean Soup served over ⅓ cup basmati rice (see recipes).

5 oz. grilled center-cut pork chop.

Southwestern Fajita, using 5 oz. lean protein (see recipes; use two small whole-wheat tortillas).

Greek Turkey Burger (see recipes) served on a lower-calorie wheat bun (approximately 80 calories per bun). Add 1 thin slice of your favorite cheese.

3 oz. sweet potato flavored with cinnamon and Splenda (optional).

5 oz. grilled fish with 1 cup lentils and 1 medium broiled tomato.

5 oz. shrimp or crawfish stir-fried with mushrooms, spinach, onions, and minced garlic in 1 tsp. olive oil and a splash of soy sauce. Serve over ⅔ cup brown rice.

Whole-wheat tortilla wrap (we prefer La Tortilla Factory) with 4 oz. turkey, chicken, or lean ham, plus 1 thin slice cheese. Dip into 4 Tbsp. hummus (or spread hummus over tortilla before wrapping). Serve with Broccoli Medley (see recipes).

Pita Pocket Sandwich: Stuff 5 oz. of your favorite lean protein (turkey, chicken, tuna, lean roast beef or ham) into a whole-wheat pita (both pockets). Add fresh spinach leaves, sliced red peppers, and a drizzle of light vinaigrette dressing.

Protein shake with 30 g whey protein (should contain no more than 4 g carbohydrates per 20 g), 1 cup skim or soy milk, 1–2 Tbsp. ground flaxseed, and ½ cup fresh or frozen berries (no sugar added). Add ice and blend.

5 whole-grain crackers or a piece of fruit.

Dinner Options

Key West Scallop Skewers (with 6–8 oz. scallops) with Spicy Sautéed Kale (see recipes).

Mixed greens salad with a splash of red wine vinaigrette to taste.

1 cup Zesty Black Beans, without rice (see recipes).

6 oz. grilled tuna or salmon.

Portobello mushrooms and red peppers, grilled or roasted with 1 tsp. olive oil and seasonings.

1 cup couscous.

Mexican-Style Lettuce Wraps, using 6 oz. chicken, 2 small whole-wheat tortillas for two wraps, and lettuce for rest (see recipes).

Shrimp Veggie Stir-Fry, using 6–8 oz. shrimp (see recipes). Serve over 1 cup basmati rice.

Mushroom and Spinach Pizza (see recipes). Add 6 oz. shrimp, turkey pepperoni, or diced chicken.

Meatloaf with a serving of Grandma's Green Bean Pie (see recipes).

6 oz. baked sweet potato flavored with ½ tsp. cinnamon and ½ tsp. vanilla extract.

Chicken and Artichokes (see recipes).

1 cup whole-wheat penne pasta with ½ Tbsp. olive oil and 1 Tbsp. Parmesan.

Mixed green salad tossed with 2 Tbsp. feta cheese and 1 Tbsp. light vinaigrette dressing.

Nirvana Kabobs with Baked Eggplant (see recipes).

1 cup Flax-Fortified Fried Rice without sirloin (see recipes).

6 oz. pork tenderloin medallions.

Cauliflower "Potato Salad" (see recipes).

1–2 cups asparagus, steamed with a splash of lemon juice and a splash of balsamic vinegar.

1 whole-wheat dinner roll.

Protein shake with 35 g whey protein (should contain no more than 6 g carbohydrates per 35 g), 1 cup skim or soy milk, 1–2 Tbsp. ground flaxseed, and fresh or frozen berries (no sugar added). Add ice and blend.

8–10 whole-grain crackers topped with 1 thin slice cheese.

Nighttime Snack Options

20 g whey protein powder blended with 1 cup skim or soy milk; add a splash of vanilla or almond extract to flavor it.

1 carton light yogurt with 2 Tbsp. sunflower seeds.

1 cup no-sugar-added ice cream (we like Blue Bell Light).

1 cup low-fat cottage cheese; add 1 Tbsp. of light yogurt or a little Splenda to flavor it.

1 cup sugar-free pudding made with skim milk; top with 1 heaping Tbsp. of whipped topping.

1 oz. cheese, any variety, rolled up with 1 oz. turkey breast.

10

Delicious Fat-Burning Recipes

It has always been my philosophy that eating for fat loss should not be boring, especially because I live in New Orleans, which is known worldwide for its fine cuisine. People are much more likely to stay on a program if the low-calorie meals and snacks they eat are flavorful and satisfying with plenty of variety. For that reason, I have worked with Chef Marc Gilberti to come up with recipes that taste so good they are absolutely guaranteed to make you forget you are trying to lose fat. Here, for your eating pleasure, are the best of my hundreds of Mackie Meals, including low-calorie versions of some of my New Orleans favorites.

Breakfast Foods

EYE-OPENING BREAKFAST BURRITOS

2 whole-wheat tortillas
cooking spray
1 red pepper, chopped
1 green pepper, chopped
½ onion, chopped

2 whole eggs and 4 egg whites, lightly beaten
½ tsp. salt
¼ tsp. cayenne pepper
¼ cup salsa

Place tortillas in oven at 250 degrees to warm. Spray pan with cooking spray and sauté peppers and onion until tender. Add egg mixture, salt, and cayenne pepper. Cook until eggs reach desired consistency (stir occasionally to keep eggs from sticking). Divide mixture onto tortillas; roll up tortillas and top with salsa.

YIELD: 2 SERVINGS

Nutrition Facts: Calories 286 ▌ Protein 18 g ▌ Carbohydrates 40 g ▌ Fat 6 g

FLAVOR-BURSTING OATMEAL

½ cup oatmeal, uncooked
1 flavored tea bag (vanilla, cinnamon apple spice, etc.)

1 tsp. trans-free butter or margarine spread (optional)
cinnamon or vanilla extract (optional)

Cook oatmeal according to package directions; place tea bag in oatmeal while cooking. When oatmeal is cooked, remove tea bag, mix in optional butter spread, cinnamon, or vanilla extract.

YIELD: 1 SERVING

Nutrition Facts: Calories 160 ▌ Protein 6 g ▌ Carbohydrates 30 g ▌ Fat 2 g

Salads and Salad Entrees

OSAKA DUCK BREAST SALAD

1 tsp. green peppercorns
1 tsp. black peppercorns
1 tsp. white peppercorns
4 duck breasts (4–6 oz. each), skinned
¼ lb. fresh spinach leaves

¼ lb. arugula
½ head romaine broken into large leaves
½ avocado, peeled and chopped
2 Tbsp. Asian-style sesame vinaigrette (any brand)

Crush the green, black, and white peppercorns. Coat duck breasts with crushed peppercorns. Sear the duck in a nonstick skillet until golden brown. Transfer duck breasts to a baking dish and bake at 350 degrees until medium-rare (approximately 20–25 minutes); set aside. In a large skillet, heat spinach, arugula, and romaine until they begin to wilt. Divide wilted lettuce leaves onto four plates. Sprinkle the avocado around the lettuce. Thinly slice the duck and arrange on top of the lettuce. Drizzle Asian sesame vinaigrette over each plate.

YIELD: 4 SERVINGS

Nutrition Facts: Calories 365 ▌ Protein 46 g ▌ Carbohydrates 7 g ▌ Fat 17 g

MEDITERRANEAN POTATO SALAD

12 new potatoes
1 Tbsp. dried basil (or 2 Tbsp.
    fresh chopped basil)
2 green onions, thinly sliced
1 tsp. black pepper

2 tsp. salt
2 Tbsp. olive oil
4 Tbsp. balsamic vinegar
2 Tbsp. lemon juice

Steam potatoes and let cool slightly; cut potatoes into quarters. In a large bowl, mix all ingredients in with potatoes. Serve chilled.

YIELD: 4 SERVINGS

Nutrition Facts: Calories 200 ▮ Protein 5 g ▮ Carbohydrates 30 g ▮ Fat 7 g

MACKIE CHICKEN SALAD

4 oz. grilled skinless chicken breast,
    sliced
½ green apple, sliced very thin
1 Tbsp. chopped walnuts

1 Tbsp. crumbled gorgonzola cheese
2 cups mixed greens
2 Tbsp. low-fat raspberry vinaigrette

Serve sliced chicken, apples, walnuts, and cheese over bed of mixed greens. Top with raspberry vinaigrette.

YIELD: 1 SERVING

Nutrition Facts: Calories 390 ▮ Protein 34 g ▮ Carbohydrates 20 g ▮ Fat 19 g

MOLLY'S FAVORITE: BLUESY SALMON SALAD

4 oz. salmon filet, grilled and
    seasoned to taste
1 Tbsp. dried cranberries

1 Tbsp. crumbled blue cheese
2 cups fresh spinach
2 Tbsp. low-fat red wine vinaigrette

Serve salmon, cranberries, and cheese over spinach. Top with vinaigrette.

YIELD: 1 SERVING

Nutrition Facts: Calories 400 ▮ Protein 34 g ▮ Carbohydrates 23 g ▮ Fat 18 g

ROCKIN' ROASTED VEGETABLE SALAD

½ cup sliced roasted zucchini

½ cup sliced roasted squash

½ cup sliced roasted eggplant

½ cup sliced roasted red and yellow peppers

½ cup sliced roasted portobello mushrooms

2 Tbsp. chopped black olives

2 cups fresh kale or mixed greens

1–2 Tbsp. balsamic vinegar

1 tsp. olive oil

Serve roasted vegetables and olives over bed of fresh kale or mixed greens. Top with balsamic vinegar and olive oil.

YIELD: 1 SERVING

Nutrition Facts: Calories 290 ▮ Protein 15 g ▮ Carbohydrates 33 g ▮ Fat 11 g

TROPICAL FRUIT MEDLEY

1 kiwifruit, sliced

½ cup fresh pineapple chunks

½ cup fresh sliced strawberries

1 Tbsp. sliced almonds

Toss all ingredients with 1 cup low-fat vanilla yogurt, or serve alone or over a bed of mixed greens.

YIELD: 1 SERVING

Nutrition Facts: Calories 265 ▮ Protein 10 g ▮ Carbohydrates 48 g ▮ Fat 4 g

MEXICAN FIESTA SALAD

½ cup canned black beans, rinsed and drained

½ cup chopped tomatoes

¼ cup chopped red onions

2 cups mixed greens

1 Tbsp. guacamole

2 Tbsp. salsa

½ toasted whole-wheat tortilla, cut into triangles

Combine black beans, tomatoes, and red onions. Serve over mixed greens and garnish with guacamole, salsa, and tortilla.

YIELD: 1 SERVING

Nutrition Facts: Calories 305 ▮ Protein 12 g ▮ Carbohydrates 55 g ▮ Fat 4 g

ATHENIAN SALAD

1 Tbsp. chopped black olives
½ cup artichoke hearts marinated in light Italian dressing
1 Tbsp. feta cheese
¼ cup finely chopped sun-dried tomatoes

2 cups arugula or mixed greens
2 Tbsp. hummus
4 toasted whole-wheat pita points

Combine black olives, artichoke hearts, feta cheese, and sun-dried tomatoes. Serve over arugula or mixed greens. Top with hummus and garnish with whole-wheat pita points.

YIELD: 1 SERVING

Nutrition Facts: Calories 360 ▮ Protein 18 g ▮ Carbohydrates 40 g ▮ Fat 15 g

ORIENT EXPRESS SALAD

4 oz. firm tofu, cubed
½ cup bean sprouts
½ cup lightly steamed carrots, cut diagonally
½ cup lightly steamed broccoli florets

2 Tbsp. mango salsa
2 cups romaine lettuce
2 Tbsp. low-fat sesame vinaigrette

Combine tofu, bean sprouts, carrots, broccoli, and salsa. Serve over romaine. Top with vinaigrette.

YIELD: 1 SERVING

Nutrition Facts: Calories 280 ▮ Protein 17 g ▮ Carbohydrates 38 g ▮ Fat 7 g

CHILLED PASTA SALAD

1 cup cooked whole-wheat bowtie or penne pasta
2 Tbsp. low-fat ranch dressing
1 Tbsp. pine nuts

¼ cup lightly steamed broccoli florets
¼ cup lightly steamed sliced carrots
6 cherry tomatoes

Toss all ingredients and serve salad chilled. Serve over bed of romaine lettuce if you wish.

YIELD: 1 SERVING

Nutrition Facts: Calories 310 ▮ Protein 18 g ▮ Carbohydrates 47 g ▮ Fat 9 g

SEARED TUNA SALAD

4 oz. tuna filet	2 cups mixed greens
cooking spray	1 Tbsp. low-sodium soy sauce
⅛ medium avocado, cubed	1 tsp. olive oil
½ mango, cubed	

Sear tuna by cooking in pan sprayed with cooking spray on medium heat. Serve tuna, avocado, and mango over mixed greens. Top with soy sauce and olive oil.

YIELD: 1 SERVING

Nutrition Facts: Calories 375 ∎ Protein 32 g ∎ Carbohydrates 25 g ∎ Fat 15 g

Vegetable Side Dishes

TOFU GUACAMOLE

1 medium avocado, ripened	4 Tbsp. chunky salsa
8 oz. extra-firm tofu, cubed	1 tsp. fresh chopped cilantro

Peel, seed, and mash the avocado. In a food processor or blender, purée the avocado and tofu. Place into a serving bowl, fold in salsa, top with cilantro, and serve immediately.

YIELD: 2 CUPS; 16 (2 TBSP.) SERVINGS

Nutrition Facts: Calories 72 ∎ Protein 3.7 g ∎ Carbohydrates 3 g ∎ Fat 5 g

OYSTER STUFFING

1½ cups chopped green onions	1 Tbsp. salt
1½ cups chopped red onions	1 Tbsp. cayenne pepper
1½ cups chopped celery	1 Tbsp. garlic powder
1½ cups chopped green pepper	1 Tbsp. fresh chopped thyme
2 Tbsp. olive oil	3 cups whole-wheat bread crumbs
½ gallon oysters in liquid	

Brown green onions, red onions, celery, and green pepper in olive oil. Add oysters and oyster liquid. Cook until vegetables are translucent. Add salt, cayenne, garlic powder, and thyme. Stir in whole-wheat bread crumbs. Bake in a casserole dish at 350 degrees for 35–40 minutes until lightly browned.

YIELD: 12 SERVINGS

Nutrition Facts: Calories 240 ▌ Protein 18 g ▌ Carbohydrates 25 g ▌ Fat 7.5 g ▌
Fiber 3 g

CAULIFLOWER "POTATO SALAD"

1 medium head cauliflower, cut in
    small florets
¼ cup light mayonnaise, such as
    Hellmann's Light
2 Tbsp. lemon juice

2 tsp. Splenda
½ tsp. dried mustard
3 green onions, chopped
2 Tbsp. chopped green pepper
salt and pepper to taste

Cook cauliflower in a large pot of boiling water for 10 minutes, until tender; drain and rinse under cold water; pat dry. In a large bowl, mix mayonnaise, lemon juice, Splenda, and mustard. Add cauliflower, green onion, and pepper. Mix well until vegetables are evenly coated with dressing. Add salt and pepper. Chill for 30 minutes for flavors to blend.

YIELD: 6 SERVINGS

Nutrition Facts: Calories 70 ▌ Protein 2.5 g ▌ Carbohydrates 7 g ▌ Fat 3.5 g

SPICY SAUTÉED KALE

1 large head kale, stems trimmed
    (or 1 package fresh kale)
2 Tbsp. olive oil
½ small red onion, chopped
1 roasted red pepper, chopped

2 Tbsp. minced garlic
3 Tbsp. red wine vinegar
1 tsp. Splenda
salt and pepper to taste

Boil kale in salted water until tender (8–10 minutes); drain and rinse under cold water, and pat dry; coarsely chop kale into large pieces. Heat olive oil in a large skillet over medium heat. Add onion and red pepper; cook 5 minutes, or until tender. Stir in garlic and allow it to brown. Add kale and cook for 3 minutes, stirring frequently. Transfer to a large bowl. Add vinegar and Splenda to skillet and cook 1 minute; pour over kale, tossing to coat. Add salt and pepper.

YIELD: 6 SERVINGS

Nutrition Facts: Calories 90 ▌ Protein 2 g ▌ Carbohydrates 9 g ▌ Fat 5 g

SIMPLE SPAGHETTI SQUASH

3-lb. spaghetti squash

Cut squash in half lengthwise and discard seeds; place squash halves, cut sides down, in a baking dish; add water to dish to a depth of ½ inch. Bake at 350 degrees for 45 minutes or until squash is tender when pierced with a fork. Remove squash from dish and cool. Scrape inside of squash with a fork to remove spaghetti-like strands.

YIELD: 1 SERVING

Nutrition Facts: Calories 45 ▌ Protein 1 g ▌ Carbohydrates 10 g ▌ Fat 0.4 g

HOT ASPARAGUS AND ARTICHOKES

Marinade
3 Tbsp. lemon juice
⅓ cup red wine vinegar
¼ cup olive oil
1 Tbsp. fresh chopped parsley
1 Tbsp. fresh chopped chives

1 large bundle fresh asparagus
  spears, trimmed
1 cup drained artichoke hearts
1 Tbsp. olive oil
½ cup fresh chopped parsley
¼ cup fresh chopped chives
2 Tbsp. chopped pimiento (optional)

Mix all marinade ingredients together. Toss asparagus and artichoke hearts in marinade; keep in a covered glass dish in the refrigerator for at least 20 minutes. Drain off as much of the marinade as possible. Heat 1 tablespoon olive oil in a large skillet; toss asparagus and artichoke hearts until heated through (about 3–4 minutes). Add parsley and chives; you can add pimiento for color at the last minute.

YIELD: 4 SERVINGS

Nutrition Facts: Calories 110 ▌ Protein 2 g ▌ Carbohydrates 10 g ▌ Fat 6 g

SPICY ROASTED SWEET POTATOES

4 tsp. coriander seeds
3 tsp. fennel seeds
2 tsp. dried oregano
1 dried red chili pepper
¾ tsp. salt

1 tsp. black peppercorns
2 garlic cloves, minced
2 Tbsp. olive oil
2 medium sweet potatoes cut into
  quarters

Grind coriander, fennel, oregano, chili pepper, salt, and pepper in a spice/coffee grinder until fine. In a small bowl, mix ground spices, garlic, and olive oil to make a paste; rub paste on sweet potatoes and place on a baking sheet. Bake at 400 degrees for 30–40 minutes until tender.

YIELD: 6 SERVINGS

Nutrition Facts: Calories 125 ▮ Protein 2 g ▮ Carbohydrates 15 g ▮ Fat 4.6 g ▮ Fiber 4 g

MASHED SWEET POTATOES

3 lb. sweet potatoes (about 7–8, depending on size)	2 Tbsp. brown sugar
	1 cup skim milk
1 Tbsp. cinnamon	2 Tbsp. olive oil

Bake sweet potatoes at 350 degrees for 50 minutes; peel, and place in bowl with cinnamon, brown sugar, and milk. Mash well, add olive oil, and mash again.

YIELD: 12 (½ CUP) SERVINGS

Nutrition Facts: Calories 160 ▮ Protein 2 g ▮ Carbohydrates 24 g ▮ Fat 2.3 g

BROCCOLI MEDLEY

2 cups fresh broccoli florets
¼ cup golden raisins or dried cranberries
⅛ cup chopped pecans (or walnuts, etc.)
½ cup sliced mushrooms (optional)
¼ to ½ cup chopped red onions (optional)

Dressing
½ cup low-fat mayonnaise
¼ cup Splenda
2 Tbsp vinegar (such as red wine or apple cider vinegar)

In a large bowl, combine broccoli, raisins or cranberries, pecans, mushrooms, and onions. Mix together dressing ingredients, adding more vinegar if needed, according to taste. Pour dressing over broccoli mixture. Refrigerate for at least 1 hour for best flavor.

YIELD: 4 SERVINGS

Nutrition Facts: Calories 130 ▮ Protein 1 g ▮ Carbohydrates 11 g ▮ Fat 9 g

ASIAN SLAW

4 cups or 1 medium head shredded cabbage	1 Tbsp. fresh chopped cilantro
1 cup matchstick carrots	4 Tbsp. low-sodium soy sauce
¼ cup thinly sliced green onions	1 Tbsp. sesame oil
¼ cup thinly sliced red onions	1 Tbsp. olive oil
	salt and pepper to taste

In large bowl, mix all ingredients together and place in refrigerator to marinate for 1 hour.

YIELD: 6 SERVINGS

Nutrition Facts: Calories 95 ∎ Protein 5 g ∎ Carbohydrates 6.5 g ∎ Fat 5 g ∎ Fiber 4.5 g

GARLIC MASHED POTATOES WITH CAULIFLOWER

3 lb. baking potatoes	4 Tbsp. trans- and saturated fat–free spread (i.e., Brummel and Brown)
1 large head garlic	
3 cups fresh cauliflower florets	
3 cups skim or low-fat milk	1½ tsp. salt
	pepper to taste

Bake potatoes at 400 degrees for 1 hour. Slice the pointed end off garlic and wrap the head in foil; put garlic, cut side up, in the oven with potatoes for 30 minutes; remove garlic, unwrap, and let cool. Cover cauliflower with milk in a large pot; bring to a boil; reduce to simmer and cook 10 minutes until tender; set aside. Cube potatoes, and smash with fork, whisk, or potato masher. Squeeze pulp out of garlic into potatoes, then add butter spread. Drain the cauliflower, setting the milk aside; add cauliflower to potatoes with approximately ¾ cup of reserved milk (more milk will make for creamier potatoes); mash until smooth. Add salt and pepper to taste.

YIELD: 12 SERVINGS

Nutrition Facts: Calories 75 ∎ Protein 3 g ∎ Carbohydrates 14 g ∎ Fat 1.8 g ∎ Fiber 2 g

Soups

CHICKEN FLORENTINE SOUP

2 lb. chicken breasts (no skin or cartilage, cut in ½-inch pieces)
2 Tbsp. olive oil
2 cups chopped onions
1 cup chopped celery
2 Tbsp. chopped garlic

8-oz. can crushed tomatoes
1 Tbsp. fresh chopped basil
1 lb. fresh spinach
salt and pepper to taste
1 Tbsp. Parmesan cheese

Sauté chicken breasts in olive oil until browned. Add onions, celery, and garlic and cook until veggies are tender. Add 3 quarts water, tomatoes, and basil; bring to a boil and simmer for 20 minutes. Add spinach and simmer for 10 minutes. Add salt and pepper to taste; garnish with Parmesan cheese.

YIELD: 6 SERVINGS

Nutrition Facts: Calories 320 ▮ Protein 47 g ▮ Carbohydrates 15 g ▮ Fat 8 g ▮ Fiber 4 g

VEGETABLE BARLEY SOUP

1 cup chopped red onions
¼ cup chopped green onions
1 cup chopped celery
2 Tbsp. olive oil
2 quarts beef broth (okay to use fat-free reduced-sodium cans such as College Hill or Swanson)
1 cup canned chopped tomatoes

2 cups broccoli cut into ½-inch pieces
2 cups cauliflower cut into ½-inch pieces
1 cup carrots cut into ¼-inch pieces
1 cup turnips cut into ½-inch pieces
1 cup barley
salt and pepper to taste

Sauté red onions, green onions, and celery in olive oil until tender. Add beef broth and tomatoes and bring to a boil. Add broccoli, cauliflower, carrots, and turnips and simmer 20 minutes; add barley and simmer another 20 minutes. Add salt and pepper to taste.

YIELD: 6 SERVINGS

Nutrition Facts: Calories 270 ▮ Protein 8 g ▮ Carbohydrates 43 g ▮ Fat 7 g ▮ Fiber 5 g

SWEET POTATO AND LEEK SOUP

1 cup chopped leeks

1 cup chopped onions

1 cup chopped celery

2 Tbsp. olive oil

2 quarts chicken broth (okay to use
fat-free reduced-sodium cans
such as College Hill or
Swanson)

1 quart skim milk

6 medium sweet potatoes, peeled,
boiled, and mashed

salt and pepper to taste

Sauté leeks, onions, and celery in olive oil. Add chicken broth and milk and bring to a boil. Add sweet potatoes and simmer 30 minutes. Add salt and pepper to taste.

YIELD: 6 SERVINGS

Nutrition Facts: Calories 270 ∎ Protein 9 g ∎ Carbohydrates 44 g ∎ Fat 6 g ∎ Fiber 5 g

BUTTERNUT SQUASH SOUP

cooking spray

2 butternut squash cut in halves

1 cup chopped onions

1 cup chopped celery

2 Tbsp. chopped garlic

2 Tbsp. olive oil

2 quarts chicken broth (okay to use
fat-free reduced-sodium cans
such as College Hill or
Swanson)

1 tsp. nutmeg

salt and pepper to taste

Spray baking sheet with cooking spray, place squash halves cut sides up, and bake at 350 degrees for 30–40 minutes until soft. Let cool, scoop out squash, and set aside. Sauté onions, celery, and garlic in olive oil. Add chicken broth, squash, and nutmeg. Using a hand mixer, blend well until smooth. Reheat. Add salt and pepper to taste.

YIELD: 6 SERVINGS

Nutrition Facts: Calories 215 ∎ Protein 2 g ∎ Carbohydrates 35 g ∎ Fat 6.5 g ∎ Fiber 4.5 g

SPLIT PEA SOUP

2 cups chopped onions
1 cup chopped celery
1 cup chopped carrots
2 Tbsp. olive oil
1 Tbsp. fresh chopped thyme
1 Tbsp. fresh chopped basil
1 gallon chicken broth (okay to use
  fat-free reduced-sodium cans
  such as College Hill or
  Swanson)

1 lb. dried split peas
1 Tbsp. garlic powder
salt and pepper to taste
1 slice whole-wheat toast, cubed

Sauté onions, celery, and carrots in olive oil until tender. Add thyme, basil, chicken broth, and split peas. Bring to a boil and add garlic powder. Simmer for 1 hour, then add salt and pepper to taste. Garnish with toast cubes.

YIELD: 6 SERVINGS

Nutrition Facts: Calories 220 ▌ Protein 10 g ▌ Carbohydrates 36 g ▌ Fat 4 g ▌ Fiber 6.5 g

CABBAGE AND RED BEAN SOUP

2 quarts chicken broth (okay to use
  fat-free reduced-sodium cans
  such as College Hill or
  Swanson)
1 medium head cabbage cut into
  ½-inch cubes
1 medium onion, chopped
1 cup chopped celery

1 cup chopped green pepper
1 Tbsp. chopped garlic
12 oz. canned chopped tomatoes
12 oz. canned kidney beans, rinsed
  and drained
½ cup fresh chopped parsley
1 Tbsp. fresh chopped basil
salt and pepper to taste

Bring chicken broth to a boil. Add cabbage, onions, celery, peppers, garlic, and tomatoes; simmer 20 minutes. Add kidney beans, parsley, basil, salt and pepper; simmer 20 minutes.

YIELD: 6 SERVINGS

Nutrition Facts: Calories 140 ▌ Protein 8 g ▌ Carbohydrates 23 g ▌ Fat 2 g ▌ Fiber 6.5 g

LENTIL SOUP

2 cups chopped onions

1 cup chopped celery

1 cup chopped carrots

2 Tbsp. olive oil

1 Tbsp. fresh chopped thyme

1 Tbsp. fresh chopped basil

1 lb. dried lentils

1 gallon chicken broth (okay to use fat-free reduced-sodium cans such as College Hill or Swanson)

1 Tbsp. garlic powder

salt and pepper to taste

Sauté onions, celery, and carrots in olive oil until tender. Add thyme, basil, lentils, and chicken broth; bring to a boil. Add garlic powder. Simmer 1 hour, then add salt and pepper to taste.

YIELD: 6 SERVINGS

Nutrition Facts: Calories 255 ▌ Protein 10 g ▌ Carbohydrates 34 g ▌ Fat 8.5 g ▌ Fiber 6 g

CORN AND CRAWFISH BISQUE

2 cups chopped red onions

1 cup chopped celery

2 Tbsp. olive oil

1 Tbsp. fresh chopped thyme

1 Tbsp. fresh chopped basil

2 quarts chicken broth (okay to use fat-free reduced-sodium cans such as College Hill or Swanson)

1 quart skim milk

12 oz. canned low-sodium whole kernel corn

12 oz. canned cream-style corn

1 Tbsp. garlic powder

3 Tbsp. cornstarch

2 Tbsp. olive oil

1 lb. cooked crawfish tails

½ cup chopped green onions

salt and pepper to taste

Sauté red onions and celery in olive oil until tender. Add thyme, basil, chicken broth, skim milk, both kinds of corn, and garlic powder; bring to a boil. Mix 3 Tbsp. water with cornstarch and add to soup to thicken; simmer 15–20 minutes. In separate skillet, heat olive oil and add crawfish and green onions; sauté 5 minutes, then add to soup. Add salt and pepper to taste.

YIELD: 6 SERVINGS

Nutrition Facts: Calories 415 ▌ Protein 22 g ▌ Carbohydrates 66 g ▌ Fat 7 g ▌ Fiber 4 g

Entrees

SHRIMP VEGGIE STIR-FRY

1 Tbsp. olive oil	⅓ cup sliced water chestnuts
4 oz. medium shrimp, peeled	1 Tbsp. minced garlic
⅓ cup sliced mushrooms	pepper to taste
⅓ cup sliced green peppers	low-sodium soy sauce to taste
⅓ cup sliced red peppers	

Heat olive oil in large skillet; add shrimp and cook while stirring for about 3 minutes; set aside. Stir-fry mushrooms, green and red peppers, water chestnuts, and garlic to desired tenderness. Add shrimp to vegetables. Season with pepper and soy sauce.

YIELD: 1 SERVING

Nutrition Facts: Calories 280 ▌ Protein 28 g ▌ Carbohydrates 20 g ▌ Fat 10 g

SOY-GLAZED SALMON

2 cups low-sodium soy sauce	½ Tbsp. chopped garlic
½ cup pineapple juice	1 Tbsp. chopped green onions
1 Tbsp. crushed red pepper flakes	2 Tbsp. cornstarch
1 Tbsp. fresh chopped ginger	4 salmon filets (4–6 oz. each)

Combine soy sauce, pineapple juice, red pepper flakes, ginger, garlic, and green onions; bring to a boil; slowly stir in cornstarch and 2 Tbsp. water. Place salmon filets in a shallow dish and cover with sauce; allow to marinate 30 minutes. Cover a baking sheet with foil; place salmon on foil and top with any remaining marinade; broil 5–7 minutes.

YIELD: 4 SERVINGS

Nutrition Facts: Calories 280 ▌ Protein 35 g ▌ Carbohydrates 13 g ▌ Fat 10 g

SALMON TERIYAKI

2 Tbsp. low-sodium soy sauce   1 tsp. minced garlic
1 Tbsp. fresh chopped ginger   2 salmon filets (4 oz. each)
½ cup minced scallions

Whisk together soy sauce, ginger, scallions, and garlic in a nonmetallic bowl. Place salmon filets in shallow dish and cover with soy-ginger sauce; allow to marinate 30 minutes. Cover a baking sheet with foil; place salmon on foil and top with any remaining marinade; broil 5–7 minutes.

YIELD: 2 SERVINGS

Nutrition Facts: Calories 200 ▮ Protein 28 g ▮ Carbohydrates 0 g ▮ Fat 9 g

VEGETARIAN KABOBS

½ cup low-fat Italian dressing   1 zucchini, thickly sliced
12 cherry tomatoes   1 green pepper cut into large pieces
1 red onion cut into large pieces   1 red pepper cut into large pieces
8 oz. fresh whole mushrooms

Heat grill. Pour dressing into a large plastic bag; add vegetables and shake to coat with dressing; allow to marinate at least 10 minutes. Soak 4 wooden skewers in water; alternate vegetables on skewers. Place skewers on grill; add extra marinade and turn skewers as needed; grill 5–8 minutes, until vegetables are tender.

YIELD: 2 SERVINGS

Nutrition Facts: Calories 175 ▮ Protein 2 g ▮ Carbohydrates 35 g ▮ Fat 3 g

GARLIC SHRIMP

8 cloves garlic, chopped   1 lb. large shrimp
⅓ cup fresh lemon juice   1 Tbsp. olive oil
1 pinch cayenne pepper   ¼ cup fresh chopped parsley

Combine garlic, lemon juice, cayenne pepper, and shrimp; marinate 1 hour in refrigerator. Heat olive oil and sauté shrimp 3 minutes on each side. Sprinkle with parsley.

YIELD: 4 SERVINGS

Nutrition Facts: Calories 145 ▮ Protein 25 g ▮ Carbohydrates 0 g ▮ Fat 5 g

GREEK TURKEY BURGERS

10 oz. package frozen chopped
spinach, thawed, drained,
and squeezed dry

1 Tbsp. lemon juice

¼ tsp. black pepper

1 large egg white, lightly beaten

¾ lb. ground turkey breast

½ cup crumbled feta cheese

¼ cup chopped fresh mint or 4 tsp.
dried mint flakes

cooking spray

4 whole-wheat hamburger buns

1 cup fresh spinach leaves

½ cup chopped tomato

Greek Yogurt Sauce

½ cup plain yogurt

½ tsp. fresh chopped dill or ⅛ tsp.
dried dill

1 tsp. minced garlic

To make Greek Yogurt Sauce, blend sauce ingredients. To make burgers, combine spinach, lemon juice, pepper, and egg white. Add ground turkey, feta, and mint, and stir well. Divide mixture and shape into 4 equal patties. Spray grill with cooking spray and grill patties about 6 minutes on each side or until done. Line bottom half of each bun with spinach leaves; top each with a patty, tomato, Greek Yogurt Sauce, and top half of bun.

YIELD: 4 SERVINGS

Nutrition Facts: Calories 400 ▮ Protein 34 g ▮ Carbohydrates 36 g ▮ Fat 14 g

HOMESTYLE "FRIED" CHICKEN

¼ cup whole-wheat bread crumbs
(white bread crumbs will work,
but whole-wheat is preferred)

1 Tbsp. grated Parmesan cheese

1 tsp. paprika

1 tsp. dried thyme

½ tsp. garlic salt

¼ tsp. cayenne pepper

⅓ cup low-fat buttermilk

4 skinless chicken breasts
(6 oz. each)

cooking spray

1 Tbsp. butter, melted

Combine bread crumbs, Parmesan, paprika, thyme, garlic salt, and cayenne in a shallow dish. Pour buttermilk into a separate shallow dish. Dip chicken in buttermilk, then dredge in bread crumb mixture. Place in baking pan coated with cooking spray and drizzle butter over chicken. Bake at 400 degrees for 40 minutes or until done.

YIELD: 4 SERVINGS

Nutrition Facts: Calories 295 ▮ Protein 44 g ▮ Carbohydrates 6.5 g ▮ Fat 9 g

EGGPLANT LASAGNA

cooking spray

2 medium eggplants, peeled and sliced ¼ inch thick

2 cups low-fat cottage cheese

2 cups fat-free ricotta cheese

1 medium onion, chopped

1 lb. very lean cooked ground beef— at least 93% lean (or ground turkey breast or vegetarian ground meat)

2 cups shredded part-skim mozzarella cheese

salt and pepper to taste

28-oz. jar pasta sauce

½ cup grated Parmesan cheese

Spray a baking dish with cooking spray. Place a layer of eggplant on bottom of dish. Then layer half of cottage cheese and ricotta cheese mixed together, then half of onions, half of ground meat, half of mozzarella, and a dash of salt and pepper. Repeat the layering, and finish with a third layer of eggplant slices. Top with jar of pasta sauce and sprinkle with Parmesan. Bake at 350 degrees for 90 minutes.

YIELD: 12 SERVINGS

Nutrition Facts: Calories 210 ▮ Protein 25 g ▮ Carbohydrates 9 g ▮ Fat 8 g

ZESTY BLACK BEANS OVER BROWN RICE

30 oz. canned black beans, rinsed and drained

4 Tbsp. sliced canned jalapeños

2 medium tomatoes, chopped

2 cloves garlic, minced

1 small green pepper, chopped

8 green onions, chopped

4 Tbsp. fresh chopped cilantro

1 Tbsp. fresh lime juice

¼ tsp lime zest

2 Tbsp. canola oil

½ tsp. salt, preferably sea salt

¼ tsp. ground cumin

3 cups steamed brown rice

Toss all ingredients thoroughly. Serve over brown rice. (Note: this recipe can also be served as a chilled black bean salad, without the rice.)

YIELD: 6 SERVINGS

Nutrition Facts: Calories 220 ▮ Protein 7.5 g ▮ Carbohydrates 43 g ▮ Fat 4.5 g

ORIENTAL-STYLE PORK CHOPS

4 center-cut pork chops (thin cut, 6 oz. each)

2 Tbsp. sesame oil

1 medium onion cut into ½-inch pieces

3 carrots, peeled and thinly sliced

10 shiitake mushrooms (soak in cold water 20 minutes if dried and cut into ¼-inch pieces)

2 cups broccoli florets

4 Tbsp. low-sodium soy sauce

5 baby corns, canned

pepper to taste

Sauté pork chops in sesame oil for 2 minutes on each side; remove from pan and set aside. Sauté onions, carrots, and mushrooms until tender. Add broccoli and soy sauce and cook 3 minutes. Add baby corn and cook 1 minute. Return pork chops to pan. Add pepper to taste.

YIELD: 4 SERVINGS

Nutrition Facts: Calories 300 ▮ Protein 38 g ▮ Carbohydrates 43 g ▮ Fat 13 g

SEARED TUNA OVER WILTED SPINACH

4 tuna steaks (4–6 oz. each)

2 Tbsp. olive oil, divided

1 Tbsp. chopped garlic

1 lb. fresh baby spinach

salt and pepper to taste

¼ Tbsp. crumbled blue cheese

In a hot skillet, sauté tuna in 1 Tbsp. olive oil for 1 minute on each side; remove from skillet and set aside. Sauté garlic in 1 Tbsp. olive oil until garlic is light brown. Add spinach; cook until spinach is wilted. Add salt and pepper to taste. Serve tuna over wilted spinach and top with blue cheese.

YIELD: 4 SERVINGS

Nutrition Facts: Calories 280 ▮ Protein 37 g ▮ Carbohydrates 10 g ▮ Fat 10 g

SOUTHWESTERN FAJITAS

1 Tbsp. olive oil

1 lb. lean flank steak, cut on a bias,
    ¼ inch thick (or chicken or
    shrimp, peeled and deveined)

1 medium onion, thinly sliced

1 green pepper, thinly sliced

4 whole-wheat tortillas

½ cup brown rice

1 tomato, chopped

½ cup canned black beans, rinsed
    and drained

¼ cup guacamole

¼ cup shredded cheddar cheese

Heat olive oil in skillet until hot. Add flank steak and cook 3 minutes or until seared. Add onions and peppers and cook 1 minute or until vegetables are slightly soft. Layer as follows on tortillas: brown rice, tomatoes, black beans, guacamole, cheese, then steak and vegetables. Fold from bottom to top.

YIELD: 4 SERVINGS

Nutrition Facts: Calories 350 ▌ Protein 29 g ▌ Carbohydrates 36 g ▌ Fat 10 g

MEDITERRANEAN SHRIMP AND PASTA

¼ cup pine nuts

½ large onion, thinly sliced

1 garlic clove, minced

1 Tbsp. plus 1 tsp. olive oil

½ cup chopped sun-dried tomatoes

6 oz. fresh baby spinach

½ cup fresh chopped basil

½ tsp. sea salt

⅛ tsp. ground black pepper

2 Tbsp. dry vermouth

2 lb. shrimp, peeled and deveined

4 cups cooked whole-wheat penne
    pasta, al dente

⅓ cup grated Parmesan cheese

Toast pine nuts in oven at 350 degrees for 10 minutes. Sauté onion and garlic in 1 Tbsp. olive oil until soft. Add sun-dried tomatoes, spinach, basil, salt, pepper, and vermouth; sauté until spinach is wilted and tomatoes are soft. Add shrimp and cook 2 minutes. Mix in pasta and remaining 1 tsp. olive oil; sauté 2 minutes. Stir in pine nuts and mix well. Add Parmesan and toss.

YIELD: 6 SERVINGS

Nutrition Facts: Calories 365 ▌ Protein 37 g ▌ Carbohydrates 31 g ▌ Fat 10 g

BUFFALO "WINGS" WITH BLUE CHEESE DIP

cooking spray

12 skinless chicken tenders (or shrimp, or crawfish)

1¼-oz. taco seasoning packet

½ cup light sour cream

2 Tbsp. crumbled blue cheese

2 Tbsp. skim or low-fat milk

4 medium celery stalks cut into 2-inch pieces

Coat a large baking sheet with cooking spray. Put chicken (or seafood) in a plastic bag, add taco seasoning, seal bag, and shake to coat. Place chicken on baking sheet and bake at 400 degrees until cooked through, about 18–20 minutes (times will vary). Stir together sour cream, blue cheese, and milk for the dip. Serve chicken with dip and celery on the side.

YIELD: 6 SERVINGS

Nutrition Facts: Calories 100 ▌ Protein 15 g ▌ Carbohydrates 2 g ▌ Fat 4 g

CHEESY MAC & CHEESE

cooking spray

2 tsp. whole-wheat flour

1⅓ cups skim milk

1 cup shredded low-fat sharp cheddar cheese

1 cup shredded low-fat mozzarella cheese, divided

½ tsp. salt

6 cups cooked whole-wheat penne or macaroni

Spray a casserole dish with cooking spray. Mix flour with ¼ cup milk, forming a paste; pour mixture into a medium saucepan and add remainder of milk. Add all of the cheddar cheese, half of the mozzarella cheese, and salt; cook over medium heat, stirring until cheese melts and mixture thickens. When the mixture is smooth and thickened, remove from heat. In a large bowl, pour cheese mixture over cooked macaroni; stir well. Transfer macaroni and cheese to casserole dish; sprinkle remaining mozzarella over the top. Bake at 400 degrees for 20–25 minutes until heated through and lightly browned.

YIELD: 6 SERVINGS

Nutrition Facts: Calories 322 ▌ Protein 19 g ▌ Carbohydrates 33 g ▌ Fat 12.5 g

MEXICAN-STYLE LETTUCE WRAPS

3 or 4 large romaine or iceberg
  lettuce leaves
4 oz. cooked skinless chicken
  breast, chopped

2 Tbsp. salsa
¼ avocado, chopped
1 Tbsp. light sour cream

Fill lettuce leaves with chicken, salsa, and avocado; add a dollop of sour cream. Roll lettuce leaves fajita-style, and enjoy.

YIELD: 1 SERVING

Nutrition Facts: Calories 215 ▮ Protein 28 g ▮ Carbohydrates 6 g ▮ Fat 9 g

HEARTY HOMEMADE CHILI

1 Tbsp. olive oil
1 cup chopped green peppers
1 cup chopped onions
1 Tbsp. minced garlic
2 Tbsp. chili powder
1 lb. ground turkey breast
16 oz. salsa
3 cups chicken broth (okay to use fat-
  free reduced-sodium cans such
  as College Hill or Swanson)

30 oz. canned kidney beans, rinsed
  and drained
1 Tbsp. tomato paste
½ cup light sour cream
½ cup chopped tomato
½ cup low-fat shredded cheddar
  cheese

Heat oil in large saucepan over medium heat. Add peppers, onions, and garlic; cook until onions are golden brown. Stir in chili powder and cook 1–2 more minutes. Add ground turkey, stirring well; cook 5–6 minutes or until meat is browned. Transfer mixture to a large pot; add salsa, chicken broth, beans, and tomato paste; bring to a simmer over medium heat. Reduce heat and simmer until chili has thickened (approximately 45 minutes). Add salt and pepper to taste. Serve with a dollop of sour cream, tomato, and cheddar cheese.

YIELD: 8 SERVINGS

Nutrition Facts: Calories 260 ▮ Protein 26 g ▮ Carbohydrates 32 g ▮ Fat 5 g

MUSHROOM AND SPINACH PIZZA

1 cup tomato sauce

4 whole-wheat pitas

1 cup fresh chopped spinach leaves

1 cup sliced mushrooms

1 cup low-fat shredded mozzarella

Spread ¼ cup sauce evenly around each pita bread. Add ¼ cup spinach, ¼ cup mushrooms, and ¼ cup cheese to each pita bread. Place on baking sheet and bake at 450 degrees for 15–20 minutes; the cheese should be melted and a little brown. Cut each pita in half.

YIELD: 8 SERVINGS

Nutrition Facts: Calories 140 ▮ Protein 7 g ▮ Carbohydrates 19 g ▮ Fat 4 g

MEATLOAF: THE ORIGINAL COMFORT FOOD!

cooking spray

2 lb. extra-lean ground beef

½ cup ground flaxseed

¼ cup whole-wheat bread crumbs

2 egg whites, lightly beaten

¼ tsp. chopped garlic

2 tsp. Dijon mustard

3 Tbsp. Parmesan cheese

1 cup chopped mushrooms

1 cup fresh chopped spinach

½ cup marinara sauce

½ cup chicken broth (okay to use fat-free reduced-sodium cans such as College Hill or Swanson)

pepper to taste

ketchup to taste

Spray two loaf pans with cooking spray. Mix all the ingredients except ketchup together thoroughly in a large bowl; divide mixture into loaf pans and top with ketchup. Bake 30–35 minutes at 350 degrees, taking care not to overcook.

YIELD: 8 SERVINGS

Nutrition Facts: Calories 302 ▮ Protein 34 g ▮ Carbohydrates 11 g ▮ Fat 13.5 g

CAJUN JAMBALAYA

1 Tbsp. canola oil

10 oz. soy sausage links, sliced into 1-inch pieces

2 cups chopped onions

1 cup chopped celery

1 cup chopped green pepper

3 small bay leaves, crushed

6 chopped garlic cloves (or 4–6 Tbsp. minced garlic)

2 Tbsp. Cajun seasoning (i.e., Tony Cachere's)

½ tsp. salt

2 cups brown rice

3 cups tomato juice

3 cups chicken broth (okay to use fat-free reduced-sodium cans such as College Hill or Swanson)

1 lb fresh chopped tomatoes or 14-oz. can chopped tomatoes

In a large pot, heat oil over medium-high heat and sauté the sausage slices until browned. Add the onions, celery, green pepper, bay leaves, garlic, Cajun seasoning, and salt. Continue to cook 10–12 minutes, stirring frequently, until the onions are browned. Stir in the rice and cook 5 more minutes, stirring occasionally. Add the tomato juice and chicken broth, stirring well, and bring to a boil. Reduce the heat to medium and simmer, covered, for 15 minutes. Add the tomatoes, stirring well. Continue cooking over low heat, covered, until rice is tender, about 1 hour.

YIELD: 6 SERVINGS

Nutrition Facts: Calories 323 ▮ Protein 22 g ▮ Carbohydrates 32 g ▮ Fat 13 g

KEY WEST SCALLOP SKEWERS

2 lb. sea scallops

½ cup fresh lime juice

1 Tbsp. olive oil

salt and pepper to taste

2 limes cut into wedges

2 Tbsp. fresh chopped cilantro

Combine scallops, lime juice, olive oil, salt, and pepper. Allow to marinate in refrigerator for at least 2 hours. Slide lime wedges and scallops onto skewers: one lime wedge for every two or three scallops. Broil 5–6 minutes, turning once. Sprinkle skewers with cilantro.

YIELD: 6 SERVINGS

Nutrition Facts: Calories 177 ▮ Protein 25 g ▮ Carbohydrates 3.5 g ▮ Fat 7 g

BAKED EGGPLANT

cooking spray

2 lb. eggplant cut into ½-inch slices

2 Tbsp. fresh lemon juice

1 tsp. oregano

salt and pepper to taste

Spray casserole dishes with cooking spray. Place one layer of eggplant slices in each dish. Bake at 425 degrees for 20 minutes or until golden brown, turning once. Arrange eggplant on serving platter and sprinkle with lemon juice. Add oregano, salt, and pepper. Serve at room temperature.

YIELD: 6 SERVINGS

Nutrition Facts: Calories 18 ▮ Protein 0.5 g ▮ Carbohydrates 4 g ▮ Fat 0 g

GRANDMA'S GREEN BEAN PIE

cooking spray

2 lb. fresh green beans, ends
   trimmed

salt to taste

½ cup finely chopped onion

1 Tbsp. minced garlic

1 Tbsp. olive oil

2 whole eggs

2 egg whites

½ cup low-fat cottage cheese

½ cup grated Parmesan cheese

pepper to taste

Spray a casserole dish with cooking spray. Boil green beans 10 minutes in a large pot of salted water. Sauté onions and garlic in olive oil until lightly browned. Drain green beans and allow to cool. Cut into 1-inch pieces; set aside. In a small bowl, mix the eggs, egg whites, and cottage cheese. Stir the green beans into the onions and garlic. Add the egg and cottage cheese mixture; add half the Parmesan cheese. Transfer to casserole dish. Sprinkle with the remaining Parmesan cheese. Bake at 300 degrees for 45 minutes or until golden brown.

YIELD: 8 SERVINGS

Nutrition Facts: Calories 90 ▮ Protein 7.5 g ▮ Carbohydrates 4 g ▮ Fat 5 g

VEGETARIAN FRITTATA

1 Tbsp. olive oil
1 small onion, finely chopped
1 cup cauliflower florets cut into
  small pieces
1 cup broccoli florets cut into small
  pieces

¼ cup fresh chopped mushrooms
4 whole eggs and 2 cartons egg
  substitute, lightly beaten
salt and pepper to taste
3 Tbsp. grated Parmesan cheese

Heat olive oil in a skillet over medium heat. Add onions, cauliflower, and broccoli and sauté until tender. Add mushrooms and cook 5 minutes. Reduce to low heat. Pour egg mixture into skillet, stirring slightly. Add salt and pepper to taste. Cook, stirring frequently, until eggs begin to firm. Lightly press egg mixture with the flat end of a spatula. Sprinkle with Parmesan cheese. Place skillet under broiler for 1 minute. Allow to cool. Use spatula to loosen edges of frittata and slide onto a plate. Cut into wedges to serve.

YIELD: 6 SERVINGS

Nutrition Facts: Calories 106 ▮ Protein 10.5 g ▮ Carbohydrates 2.5 g ▮ Fat 6 g

CHICKEN AND ARTICHOKES

1 Tbsp. olive oil
4 boneless, skinless chicken breasts
  (6 oz. each)
¼ cup whole-wheat baking mix
12-oz. jar marinated artichokes,
  drained, liquid reserved
1 small yellow onion, chopped

8 oz. sliced mushrooms
3 Tbsp. minced garlic
½ tsp. dried oregano
½ tsp. dried rosemary
½ cup white wine
salt and pepper to taste

Heat olive oil in a large skillet over medium heat. Coat chicken with baking mix. Sauté chicken until lightly browned, turning once; transfer to a baking dish. Add artichoke liquid to skillet; cook 5 minutes, or until liquid thickens. Add onions, mushrooms, garlic, oregano, and rosemary; cook 5 minutes, until onions are tender. Stir in artichokes and wine. Pour mixture over chicken, cover, and bake at 350 degrees for 40 minutes, until chicken is tender and cooked thoroughly.

YIELD: 4 SERVINGS

Nutrition Facts: Calories 250 ▮ Protein 30 g ▮ Carbohydrates 17 g ▮ Fat 7 g

NIRVANA KABOBS

¾ cup plain yogurt

1 Tbsp. minced ginger

1 Tbsp. fresh chopped cilantro

2 tsp. chili powder

1 tsp. ground coriander

1 tsp. dried mint

4 boneless, skinless chicken breasts
(6 oz. each) cut into 1-inch
cubes

1 green pepper cut into large pieces

1 red pepper cut into large pieces

1 Tbsp. olive oil

½ tsp. salt

lime wedges

Combine yogurt, ginger, cilantro, chili powder, coriander, and mint in a shallow bowl. Add chicken and marinate in refrigerator at least 4 hours. Soak four wooden skewers in water. Thread chicken and green and red peppers onto skewers. Place on a baking sheet. Drizzle with olive oil and sprinkle with salt. Bake at 350 degrees for 30 minutes, turning once, until golden brown and cooked through. Garnish with lime wedges.

YIELD: 4 SERVINGS

Nutrition Facts: Calories 202 ▮ Protein 32 g ▮ Carbohydrates 5 g ▮ Fat 6 g

TURKEY CUTLETS

1 Tbsp. olive oil

1 lb. turkey cutlets

salt and pepper to taste

1 zucchini cut into large pieces

1 yellow squash cut into large
pieces

1 red pepper cut into large pieces

8 oz. sliced mushrooms

2 Tbsp. minced garlic

½ cup canned tomato puree

1 tsp. dried basil

¼ tsp. Splenda

Heat olive oil in a saucepan over medium heat. Sprinkle turkey cutlets with salt and pepper; cook 3 minutes per side, until lightly golden. Transfer to plate. Add zucchini, squash, and red pepper; cook 5 minutes, stirring occasionally to prevent sticking. Stir in mushrooms, garlic, tomato puree, basil, and Splenda. Bring to a boil. Cover, reduce heat, and cook 5 minutes. Add turkey to skillet. Cook, uncovered, 2–3 minutes, until turkey is heated through.

YIELD: 4 SERVINGS

Nutrition Facts: Calories 240 ▮ Protein 28 g ▮ Carbohydrates 7.5 g ▮ Fat 11 g

ROYAL BOK CHOY

2 Tbsp. low-sodium soy sauce

1 tsp. Splenda

1 Tbsp. canola oil

1 tsp. sesame oil

2 cups bok choy, cut crosswise into
2-inch pieces

4 green onions, finely chopped

3 Tbsp. minced garlic

1 Tbsp. cayenne pepper

2 Tbsp. chopped cashews

Mix soy sauce, 2 Tbsp. water, and Splenda in a small bowl; set aside. In a large skillet, heat canola and sesame oils over medium-high heat. Add bok choy, green onions, garlic, soy sauce mixture, and cayenne pepper. Sauté until bok choy starts to wilt, about 3 minutes. Stir in cashews.

YIELD: 4 SERVINGS

Nutrition Facts: Calories 115 ∥ Protein 5.5 g ∥ Carbohydrates 7 g ∥ Fat 7 g

PENNE PRIMAVERA WITH GOAT CHEESE

½ cup fresh asparagus, trimmed and
cut into 1-inch pieces

8 cherry tomatoes, halved

1 Tbsp. fresh chopped basil

1 Tbsp. minced garlic

1 cup cooked penne pasta

2 oz. feta cheese

salt and pepper to taste

Microwave asparagus on high with 2 Tbsp. water until slightly tender, about 3 minutes. In a large bowl, toss asparagus, tomatoes, basil, and garlic. Toss pasta with asparagus/tomato mixture. Add feta cheese and stir well. Add salt and pepper to taste. Refrigerate at least 20 minutes.

YIELD: 2 SERVINGS

Nutrition Facts: Calories 195 ∥ Protein 7 g ∥ Carbohydrates 25 g ∥ Fat 7.5 g

SICILIAN ZITI

cooking spray

1 cup chopped broccoli

½ cup chopped green pepper

¼ cup chopped mushrooms

2 Tbsp. minced garlic

14-oz. can low-sodium diced
tomatoes

1 tsp. dried basil

1 tsp. dried oregano

½ tsp. black pepper

1 cup cooked whole-wheat ziti or
penne pasta

½ cup part-skim mozzarella cheese

½ cup Parmesan cheese

Spray skillet with nonstick cooking spray and sauté broccoli and green peppers over medium heat for 5 minutes. Add mushrooms and garlic and cook an additional 5 minutes. Add tomatoes, basil, oregano, and pepper. Mix well. Cook over low heat 3–5 minutes. Toss the vegetables, pasta, and mozzarella cheese in a large mixing bowl. Transfer to a casserole dish sprayed with cooking spray, and top with Parmesan cheese. Bake at 375 degrees for 30 minutes, or until hot and bubbly.

YIELD: 2 SERVINGS

Nutrition Facts: Calories 353 ▌ Protein 17 g ▌ Carbohydrates 42 g ▌ Fat 13 g

OLD SCHOOL SLOPPY JOES

cooking spray	1 medium green pepper, chopped
12 oz. ground beef, at least 94% lean	10.5-oz. can low-sodium tomato soup
1 medium onion, chopped	2 whole-wheat hamburger buns

In a saucepan sprayed with nonstick cooking spray, brown meat with onions and green peppers. Add tomato soup and mix well. Simmer on low heat for 10 minutes. Place ⅔ cup of the mixture on a hamburger bun. Any extra can be frozen.

YIELD: 2 SERVINGS

Nutrition Facts: Calories 381 ▌ Protein 40 g ▌ Carbohydrates 35 g ▌ Fat 9 g

CHP WRAP (CHICKEN, HUMMUS, AND PEPPERS)

2 whole-wheat tortillas	2 cups fresh spinach leaves, trimmed
4 Tbsp. hummus	½ cup chopped tomatoes
2 boneless, skinless chicken breasts (6 oz. each), cooked (roasted, grilled, baked, or broiled) and then sliced	2 roasted red peppers, sliced

Warm tortillas in a 200-degree oven. Spread 2 Tbsp. hummus on each tortilla. Layer sliced chicken breast on top of hummus. Top with spinach leaves, tomatoes, and roasted red peppers. Wrap and serve.

YIELD: 2 SERVINGS

Nutrition Facts: Calories 335 ▌ Protein 35 g ▌ Carbohydrates 45 g ▌ Fat 6 g

FLAX-FORTIFIED FRIED RICE WITH SIRLOIN

½ cup brown rice
¼ cup flaxseeds
1 Tbsp. canola oil
2 eggs plus 2 egg whites, beaten
½ cup chopped red peppers
½ cup carrots, sliced diagonally

2 green onions cut into ¼-inch pieces
4 oz. cooked lean sirloin cut into bite-size pieces (or shrimp or chicken)
2 Tbsp. low-sodium soy sauce
½ tsp. sesame oil

Boil rice according to package directions; allow to cool to room temperature. Toast flaxseeds in oven at 350 degrees for 10–12 minutes. Heat canola oil in a large nonstick skillet over medium heat. Add eggs, frying for 1 minute. Add rice, stirring well. Add red peppers, carrots, and onions, stirring frequently until tender. Add sirloin, soy sauce, sesame oil, and toasted flaxseeds. Cover and cook on low heat 5 minutes.

YIELD: 4 SERVINGS

Nutrition Facts: Calories 210 ▮ Protein 16 g ▮ Carbohydrates 20 g ▮ Fat 7.5 g

Desserts

MELT-IN-YOUR-MOUTH FRUIT KABOBS

2 cups sliced strawberries
6 kiwifruits, peeled and quartered lengthwise
4 large pears, chopped into bite-size pieces
½ fresh pineapple cut into chunks

Glaze
½ cup sugar-free maple syrup
1 Tbsp. cinnamon
1 Tbsp. vanilla extract
3 Tbsp. trans- and saturated fat–free spread (i.e., Brummel and Brown)

Place strawberries, kiwifruit, pears, and pineapple onto skewers and grill about 2 minutes on each side, or until browned. Mix glaze ingredients together and warm on the stove. Drizzle over kabobs.

YIELD: 6 SKEWERS (APPROXIMATELY)

Nutrition Facts: Calories 30 ▮ Protein 0 g ▮ Carbohydrates 4g ▮ Fat 0 g

FUDGY MINT BROWNIES

butter-flavored cooking spray	1 tsp. peppermint extract
¾ cup light silken tofu, drained	1¼ cups cake flour
¼ cup light corn syrup	⅔ cup fructose
½ cup unsweetened cocoa powder	½ tsp. salt
2 Tbsp. almond oil	½ tsp. baking powder
1 Tbsp. vanilla extract	powdered sugar

Spray a sheet cake pan with cooking spray. In a food processor, blend tofu, corn syrup, cocoa powder, almond oil, vanilla and peppermint extracts until smooth. In a large mixing bowl, combine flour, fructose, salt, and baking powder. Add mixture from food processor and stir well to remove lumps. Pour into cake pan and bake 25–35 minutes or until a toothpick inserted in the center comes out clean. Cool brownies in pan, then dust with powdered sugar.

YIELD: 12 SERVINGS

Nutrition Facts: Calories 120 ▮ Protein 2.5 g ▮ Carbohydrates 23 g ▮ Fat 2.5 g

CHOCOLATE PEANUT BUTTER PIE

nonstick cooking spray	2 Tbsp. trans- and saturated fat–free
6 cups fat-free, sugar-free vanilla	spread (i.e., Brummel and
frozen yogurt	Brown), melted
1 cup finely crushed graham	2 Tbsp. light corn syrup
crackers	¼ cup chocolate syrup
¼ cup unsweetened cocoa powder	1½ Tbsp. peanut butter
¼ cup powdered sugar	1 tsp. skim milk

Spray a 9-inch pie plate with cooking spray. Allow frozen yogurt to become soft but not melted or runny. In a medium bowl, mix graham cracker crumbs with cocoa powder and powdered sugar. Add melted butter and corn syrup and stir. The crumbs should be sticky but not soggy. Spoon into pie plate. Using a piece of waxed paper, press the crumbs to evenly cover bottom and sides of pie plate. In a small bowl, stir chocolate syrup into peanut butter until all lumps are removed; the mixture should be like a paste. Spread about two-thirds of mixture evenly over bottom of crust. Set the other one-third aside. Spoon softened frozen yogurt on top of peanut butter mixture in pie plate in an even mound. When pie plate is full, smooth top with spatula. If yogurt seems soft or runny, return pie to freezer to harden before next step. Add milk to left-over chocolate/peanut butter mixture and stir until smooth. Using a spoon, drizzle mixture over top of pie in a swirling motion. If mixture is too thick to drizzle, add more milk, a drop at a time, stirring until it reaches desired consistency. Put pie in freezer.

YIELD: 8 SERVINGS

Nutrition Facts: Calories 233 ▮ Protein 8 g ▮ Carbohydrates 39 g ▮ Fat 5 g

YOGURT PARFAIT

1 cup light vanilla yogurt
¼ cup blackberries
¼ cup blueberries

¼ cup strawberries
2 Tbsp. low-fat granola

Alternate layers of yogurt with berries. Top with granola and serve.

YIELD: 1 SERVING

Nutrition Facts: Calories 201 ▮ Protein 9 g ▮ Carbohydrates 38.5 g ▮ Fat 1 g

CHOCOLATE MILKSHAKE

3 oz. silken tofu
1 cup soy milk
1 packet Splenda

2 Tbsp. cocoa
¼ cup Cool Whip
1 Tbsp. chocolate chips/sprinkles

Place tofu, soy milk, Splenda, and cocoa in blender and blend thoroughly. Pour in dessert glass and top with Cool Whip and chocolate chips/sprinkles.

YIELD: 1 SERVING

Nutrition Facts: Calories 295 ▮ Protein 10 g ▮ Carbohydrates 38 g ▮ Fat 13 g

REFRESHING YOGURT PIE

1 cup Cool Whip
3 cups light flavored yogurt (i.e.,
    lemon, strawberry, peach)

1 graham cracker pie crust

In large bowl, mix Cool Whip and yogurt together. Pour mixture into graham cracker pie crust and place into freezer. Serve frozen.

YIELD: 8 SERVINGS

Nutrition Facts: Calories 235 ▮ Protein 10 g ▮ Carbohydrates 27 g ▮ Fat 10 g

CHOCOLATE PEANUT BUTTER DROPS

1 oz. unsweetened chocolate
¼ cup natural peanut butter
2 Tbsp. trans- and saturated fat–free
    spread (i.e., Brummel and
    Brown)

⅓ cup low-fat ricotta cheese
3–4 packets Splenda
1 tsp. vanilla

Melt chocolate, peanut butter, and butter-style spread in the microwave. Stir well. Add ricotta, Splenda, and vanilla, mixing well. Drop by table-spoon onto waxed paper. Chill until firm.

YIELD: 12 SERVINGS

Nutrition Facts: Calories 60 ▮ Protein 2.2 g ▮ Carbohydrates 1.2 g ▮ Fat 5 g

THE PERFECT COOKIE

¾ cup trans- and saturated fat–free
    spread (i.e., Brummel and
    Brown)
1½ cups granulated fructose
¾ cup ground flaxseed
2 eggs

1 tsp. vanilla
1 cup whole-wheat flour
1 tsp. baking soda
1 tsp. ground cinnamon
½ tsp. salt (optional)
3 cups uncooked oats

In a large bowl, beat butter-style spread and fructose until creamy. Blend in flaxseed. Add eggs and vanilla extract; beat well. Add whole-wheat flour, baking soda, cinnamon, and salt; mix well. Add oats; mix well. Drop dough by rounded tablespoons onto ungreased baking sheets. Bake at 350 degrees for 8–10 minutes for a chewy cookie or 10–12 minutes for a crisp cookie. Cool 1 minute on baking sheets. Remove to wire rack; cool completely. Store tightly covered.

YIELD: 4 DOZEN

Nutrition Facts (1 cookie): Calories 70 ▮ Protein 2 g ▮ Carbohydrates 12 g ▮ Fat 2.4 g ▮ Fiber 1.5 g

WHOLE-WHEAT BLUEBERRY NUT BREAD

½ cup trans- and saturated fat–free spread (i.e., Brummel and Brown)

1 cup Splenda

2 eggs

1 tsp. vanilla extract

2 cups sifted whole-wheat flour

1 tsp. baking soda

½ tsp. salt

1 cup blueberries

½ cup chopped walnuts

cooking spray

In a large bowl, beat butter substitute and Splenda until creamy. Add eggs and vanilla extract; mix well. Add whole-wheat flour, baking soda, and salt; mix well. Stir in blueberries and walnuts. Spray a loaf pan with cooking spray. Pour mixture into loaf pan. Bake at 350 degrees for 1 hour.

YIELD: 12 SLICES

Nutrition Facts: Calories 145 ▮ Protein 4 g ▮ Carbohydrates 16 g ▮ Fat 7 g

11

Six Supplements for Fat Loss

There is a great deal of confusion out there about what kinds of supplements you should take when trying to increase metabolic efficiency and lose fat. Some people fall victim to every new weight-loss powder, pill, or fad, sometimes spending hundreds of dollars a month on products that might be useless or downright harmful. Others might be taking some of the right supplements but don't know how much to take or when to take them. With some supplements, timing is everything.

I don't feel that supplementation should be complicated or overly expensive. When clients sign up for my Fat-Burning Metabolic Fitness Plan, I explain to them that they should take supplements in two basic categories if they want to lose fat and improve their health:

1. A good multivitamin/mineral with antioxidants
2. Supplements that increase metabolism and effectively burn fat during exercise

Always Take a Good Multivitamin/Mineral

I can't emphasize enough how simply taking a high-quality multivitamin/mineral supplement can help promote general health, a stronger immune system, and good metabolic function. When buying a multivitamin/mineral, always read the label to see what you are getting. Many products provide a wide spectrum of nutrients, but I suggest taking one that includes the following:

Nutrient	Amount
Vitamin A (as beta-carotene)	10,000 IU
Vitamin C (as ascorbic acid)	600 mg
Vitamin D	400 IU
Vitamin E	200 IU
Vitamin K	60 mcg
Thiamin	60 mg
Riboflavin	30 mg
Niacin	60 mg
Vitamin B6	60 mg
Folic acid	800 mcg
Vitamin B12	800 mcg
Biotin	600 mcg
Pantothenic acid	100 mg
Calcium (as calcium carbonate and calcium citrate)	1,000 mg
Iron	18 mg
Iodine	300 mcg
Magnesium (aspartate or glycenate)	300 mg
Zinc (monomethionine)	15 mg
Selenium	100 mcg
Copper	1.5 mg
Manganese	15 mg
Chromium (as chromium picolinate)	200 mcg
Molybdenum	25 mcg

I take the vitamins formulated by Dr. Michael Murray. They are made by a highly respected company called Natural Factors and come in special formulations for men and women. Other leading companies that make excellent multivitamin/mineral supplements are Enzymatic Therapy, NOW, Solaray, and Solgar. The staff at your local health food store will be able to assist you in picking a good brand.

Learn How Supplements Can Increase Fat Loss

Over the last three decades I have found that certain types of minerals, antioxidants, and amino acids can increase metabolic function and burn fat more efficiently. As part of my Fat-Burning Metabolic Fitness Plan, I suggest that clients take my Metabolic Fitness Six Fat-Loss Supplements. The supplements described below will not only help you take off the fat, but some of them also improve heart health, improve insulin response, and lower blood pressure and cholesterol.

The Metabolic Fitness Six

1. Calcium. Most people think of calcium as something you should take to minimize bone loss with the onset of andropause or menopause, and indeed this is true. But calcium also has many other health benefits, including the ability to aid in fat reduction. An article in the *Journal of Nutritional Biochemistry,* which evaluated five clinical studies involving 780 women in their thirties, fifties, and eighties, showed that taking 1,000 mg calcium daily was associated with as much as an 8 kg (17.6 pounds) loss in body weight over four years.

A random analysis of forty-three other studies showed that 1,000 mg calcium a day over a period of two weeks led to a significant reduction in blood pressure. Calcium also lowers serum cholesterol. A recent study conducted on 223 healthy postmenopausal women showed that taking 1,000 mg calcium per day produced a 7 percent increase in HDL and a 6 percent decrease in LDL.

Early in life, taking calcium carbonate is all right because your body is able to readily absorb it. But as you move into your fifties, you should switch over to calcium citrate, which is twice as easy to absorb. You need stomach acid to absorb calcium, and as you get older your levels of stomach acid may drop. This is one of the reasons why taking Tums, which is an acid neutralizer, is not the best way to get your calcium. I suggest taking 1,000 to 1,500 mg calcium citrate with meals, as recommended by your physician.

Since calcium needs vitamin D to be absorbed, make sure you are getting 400–600 mg of D daily. Check your multiple vitamin for sufficient levels of vitamin D.

2. Magnesium. Taking magnesium will greatly enhance the effects of calcium. Magnesium is an essential partner in many enzymatic reactions that govern neuromuscular function and the maintenance of cardiovascular tone. Recent studies are beginning to find a correlation between magnesium and fat loss. People who are obese have very low levels of magnesium as compared to those with a normal body weight. If you have type 2 diabetes, taking magnesium helps to decrease insulin resistance.

Magnesium has the ability to increase calcium's effectiveness in lowering blood pressure and serum cholesterol levels. I suggest taking 450 mg magnesium glycinate or aspartate (not in combination with calcium but as a separate supplement) before bedtime.

If you have a kidney disorder, you may need to check with your doctor before supplementing with magnesium.

3. Chromium Picolinate. This supplement helps to burn fat because it increases the body's sensitivity to glucose. I usually recommend that clients take 200 mcg twice daily with a meal while they are on my program. I usually see the greatest results from this supplement after six weeks. Any good multiple vitamin should include 200 mcg chromium picolinate, so please read your vitamin/mineral label before you take an additional dose. After two months, you can drop down to a 200 mcg maintenance dose. A study from the University of Vermont also shows that chromium picolinate significantly improves glucose sensitivity in diabetics. For this reason, if you have diabetes or are hypoglycemic, speak with your doctor before taking this supplement. This is especially crucial if you are taking insulin, because chromium picolinate could change your body's insulin requirements.

4. Coenzyme Q10. Besides being a powerful antioxidant, coenzyme Q10 improves metabolic efficiency and endurance when taken before an exercise session, helps to decrease insulin resistance, and doubles your body's ability to eliminate metabolic toxins. I recommend 50 mg for women and 100 mg for men, which should be taken before cardiovascular exercise or interval training. Taking this supplement with a snack containing fat (like a small handful of nuts or a tablespoon of peanut butter) will help your body to absorb it.

There has been extensive research in the United States and Japan regarding the treatment of cardiovascular disease with coenzyme Q10. Taking this supplement will certainly help to keep your heart healthy. Most recently, coenzyme Q10 has been shown to be effective in treating high-risk breast cancer. Since this supplement is an immune function enhancer, it could also be used to decrease cancer risk.

5. Acetyl-L-Carnitine. I always use acytyl-L-carnitine in conjunction with coenzyme Q10 because this combination enhances mitochondrial function. I have found that most people who have become overfat are not only insulin resistant and glucose intolerant but have impaired mitochondrial function. In essence, the mitochondria in their cells—the little fat-burning furnaces—are no longer able to work efficiently. When I have women take

500 mg acetyl-L-carnitine and men 1,000 mg, along with their coenzyme Q10, I see a steady increase in metabolic efficiency and exercise endurance, as well as an increase in fat loss. Take this supplement before aerobic exercise or interval training.

6. Green Tea Extract. This extract, 200 to 300 mg taken 30 to 45 minutes before a workout, will increase your fat-burning efficiency. A study published in the *American Journal of Clinical Nutrition* showed that "green tea extract has thermogenic properties and promotes fat oxidation beyond that explained by its caffeine content." Other studies have shown that green tea causes fat loss in three ways:

1. The catechin polyphenols in green tea inhibit the action of the enzyme in the body that breaks down norepinephrine, extending that hormone's life in the body as a fat burner.
2. Green tea partially inhibits the action of lipase in the stomach and intestines. Lipase is a soap-like enzyme responsible for changing the fats we eat into a form the body can absorb.
3. Green tea helps insulin to more effectively remove sugar from the bloodstream, keeping blood sugar levels more consistent.

A recent article in *Nutrition* showed that green tea can protect against gastritis (inflammation of the mucous membrane of the stomach) and stomach cancer.

Other Supplements That Show Promise

There are three other supplements that have been receiving so much attention in the press lately that I would be remiss in not mentioning them here.

The first is alpha-lipoic acid, a powerful antioxidant that is both water and fat soluble. This supplement has been shown to be highly effective in reducing free radicals in the body. Most important, at appropriate doses it has been found to have a significant effect on increasing insulin sensitivity in people suffering from type 2 diabetes.

The second is conjugated linoleic acid. Some studies have shown that this supplement promotes fat loss, preserves and even increases lean muscle, increases bone density, and increases immune function. For these reasons, it has been marketed to bodybuilders as a safe alternative to steroids. While the jury is still out on whether this supplement will live up to its initial claims in further clinical trials, I felt it was worth mentioning here.

The third supplement that I recommend for fat loss is omega-3. The latest research shows that getting enough omega-3 in the diet helps decrease body fat and increase lean muscle. I suggest taking 5 g per day either in the form of fish oil capsules, flaxseed oil, and/or as ground flaxseed sprinkled on cereal or a salad.

PART THREE

The Fat-Burning Metabolic Fitness Exercise Plan

12

Exercise Burns Fat
and Benefits Health

Although most people would agree that exercise is important, the latest government report says that seven in ten adults don't exercise regularly and nearly four in ten aren't physically active at all. What's more, the figures haven't changed over the last five years, despite the warnings that a couch potato lifestyle can lead to health problems. Unfortunately, most people probably wouldn't be able to list more than a few benefits of exercise. They might say, "It makes you look good," "It helps you to lose weight," or "Exercise makes your heart stronger."

Ten Significant Benefits of Exercise

The benefits of physical activity are more far-reaching than people realize. Exercising is one of the easiest and most cost-effective ways of improving all kinds of medical conditions such as hypertension, heart disease, type 2 diabetes, thyroid problems, and depression. While it is best to follow a specific program, such as the one described in this book, studies have shown that even ten minutes a day of aerobic activities like walking or riding a bicycle can have a positive effect on health. That's how sensitive the body is to exercising.

To help you understand what you might receive from the Fat-Burning Metabolic Fitness Exercise Plan described in this book, here are ten significant benefits of exercise.

Benefit 1: Reduces Fat, Not Just Pounds

As we have seen, scale weight can be deceiving. The goal of any good weight-loss program should be to lose fat, not lean muscle tissue. While most people connect weight loss with going on a calorically restrictive diet, few realize that exercise is a powerful tool for taking off the weight. A recent article in the *Journal of Nutritional Biochemistry* reported that while dieting did take off the pounds, exercising was more effective at reducing pounds of body fat: "Although total fat decreased in both weight loss groups (exercise vs. diet), the average reduction was greater in the exercise-induced weight loss group than in the diet-induced weight loss group." Exercise also preserved and even increased lean muscle tissue, whereas dieting alone tended to reduce lean muscle to a certain degree.

The ideal presented in this article, which I also recommend in this book, is to exercise appropriately and restrict your daily caloric intake. This is the winning combination for increasing metabolism, resulting in the greatest amount of fat loss in the shortest period of time.

Benefit 2: Improves Blood Profile

According to a recent survey of studies conducted by the Human Nutrition Program, regular exercise also improves blood chemistry on many levels, from the lipid profile, to levels of hormones, to amounts of glucose and insulin.

- Exercise lowers total cholesterol and increases levels of HDL (good cholesterol).
- Exercise decreases the amount of leptin, a hormone that plays a role in regulating body fat and energy, in your bloodstream. The more leptin present, the higher your body fat.
- Exercise stimulates the production of epinephrine, a potent hormone that stimulates LPL lipase, an enzyme that catalyzes the release of free fatty acids from adipose tissues. The more epinephrine and lipase, the lower your body fat.
- Exercise decreases levels of insulin in the blood, which in turn decrease the amount of glucose present.

While dieting alone can cause some of these changes in blood chemistry, regular exercise along with dieting increases all of these benefits. It is important to remember that a woman's blood chemistry responds best to lower- to moderate-intensity exercise and a man's blood chemistry to moderate to higher levels of intensity. An article in the *Journal of Nutritional Biochemistry* that studied the cholesterol levels of male cyclists showed the effectiveness of prolonged high-intensity cardiovascular exercise in decreasing levels of LDL (bad cholesterol) and increasing levels of HDL (good cholesterol).

Benefit 3: Reduces Blood Pressure

Hypertension is so prevalent in the United States that the National Heart, Lung, and Blood Institute of the National Institute of Health has come up with a whole new set of guidelines for those who may be at risk for developing high blood pressure. There are now three categories:

1. Normal—the systolic pressure is less than 120 and the diastolic is less than 80.
2. Prehypertension—the systolic range is 120–139 and the diastolic range is 80–89.
3. Hypertension—the systolic number is greater than 139 and the diastolic is greater than 89.

Since blood pressure increases steadily with age, getting it under control and keeping it under control is crucial. A number of studies have shown that the mortality from heart attacks, strokes, and other vascular diseases increases progressively as blood pressure levels rise. The Framingham Heart Study suggests that even people who have normal blood pressure at age fifty-five still have a 90 percent chance of developing high blood pressure if lifestyle choices that prevent these increases are ignored. When coupled with fat loss from an appropriate food program, such as the one described in this book, regular and appropriate exercise is one of the lifestyle changes that has been shown to decrease hypertension significantly.

Benefit 4: Increases Elasticity of Major Arteries

Aging in adults is associated with a marked decline in the flexibility of the large elastic arteries that promote circulation in the chest region—in other words, those huge arteries that help your heart to circulate blood. The more sedentary the individual, the greater the stiffness of these arteries and the less efficient cardiac circulation becomes. Even healthy adults can suffer from this condition. Studies have shown, however, that regular exercise appears to minimize age-related changes in the elastin and collagen that make up the artery walls, enabling them to retain their flexibility.

Benefit 5: Protects against Breast Cancer

A recent study published by the *Journal of the American Medical Association* reported that even modest levels of physical activity, coupled with a reduced caloric intake to help lose body fat, decreased a woman's chances of having breast cancer. This was one of the largest studies of its kind involving 74,000 women between fifty and seventy-nine years old. An important point was that this exercise did not have to be intense: "While longer duration of physical activity provides the greatest protective benefit, such activity need not be strenuous." This is in keeping with what I have written about women benefiting most from low- to moderate-intensity exercise.

Benefit 6: Protects against Sarcopenia (Muscle Wasting)

Most people believe that a significant loss of muscle mass (sarcopenia) is inevitable with age, leading to decreased strength, mobility, and flexibility. This is not so. According to a recent article published by the *Journal of the American Academy of Orthopaedic Surgeons,* most age-related changes in muscle can be reversed through an appropriate exercise program incorporating both aerobic and resistance/strength training (working with weights or objects that you have to push against).

Individuals suffering from sarcopenia experience a significant decrease in energy levels and strength. I have discussed this topic with a seventy-year-old mentor of mine who is a retired doctor. Since my friend was involved in sports medicine, we used to discuss whether the nutrient creatine could be beneficial in the treatment of sarcopenia and in the preservation of muscle mass when you exercise. One day he said to me, "You know, I really need to start exercising."

So, at age seventy this very learned doctor made the decision that he was going to deal with his increasing waistline. He joined the Mackie Shilstone Pro Spa and began to do the Fat-Burning Metabolic Fitness Plan just three days a week (days 1, 3, and 5). He did one ten-minute circuit and fifty minutes on a recumbent bike.

Over the last five years he has experienced a dramatic increase in his lean muscle mass, a drop in his waist measurement, a significant increase in his metabolism, and he has become more active in his daily life. For me, he is a testimony to the fact that it's never too late to start exercise, and it's never too late to preserve lean muscle mass. To this day he is still doing this workout three days a week.

Benefit 7: Combats Erectile Dysfunction

A recent study of over 31,000 men between the ages of fifty-three and ninety showed that exercise delayed the onset of erectile dysfunction with age and improved sexual performance in those who already suffered from this problem. This research project, conducted by the Harvard School of Public Health, found that an average of one-third of test subjects reported problems getting and keeping an erection. Most of the men studied said that they had few problems before age fifty, but 26 percent had difficulty between ages fifty and fifty-nine; 40 percent between ages sixty and sixty-nine; and 61 percent over age seventy. Men who watched more than twenty hours of television per week, consumed too much alcohol, smoked, were overweight, had diabetes, had a previous stroke, or took antidepressants or beta-blockers had the most problems with ED.

One of the most interesting conclusions of this study was the connection between overall cardiovascular health and the ability to sustain an erection. ED could even be viewed as an early warning system that something was seriously wrong with the body's vascular system and heart health.

Men who did the equivalent of three hours per week of high-intensity cardiovascular exercise such as running or playing tennis had a 30 percent lower risk of erectile dysfunction. It is important to note that researchers stress high-intensity exercise in combating ED. In my program, I too have found that men get greater cardiovascular benefits and lose fat more effectively when their IIT (instinctive intensity training) levels are on the higher side of the scale.

Benefit 8: Protects Postmenopausal Women from Fat Gain and Loss of Lean Muscle

Lately, there has been a great deal of controversy over the safety of hormone replacement therapy. The major study designed by the Women's Health Initiative was stopped midway because some participants taking HRT developed higher incidences of breast cancer and heart disease.

The main argument in favor of HRT has been that it has the ability to help postmenopausal women conserve lean muscle and avoid gaining body fat. The American College of Sports Medicine published an article in which researchers were seeking an alternative solution to taking HRT to maintain a healthy body composition. Four groups of women participated in a resistance exercise program:

1. No exercise, no HRT
2. No exercise, HRT
3. Exercise, HRT
4. Exercise, no HRT

At the end of one year, researchers discovered that the group of women who exercised and did not take HRT did better than the nonexercise HRT group and did as well or a little better than the group that exercised and took HRT. They concluded that resistance exercise was just as effective for menopausal women in keeping off body fat as taking HRT.

Benefit 9: Protects against Osteoporosis

Most people have heard that exercise helps protect against bone loss, especially as men and women reach menopause or andropause. But many do not know that the type of exercise determines the level of bone health.

In order to not only maintain bone density but to build it, you need to do exercises that "overload" the bone, giving it something to lift or push against that forces it to work at a higher level than it experiences in your day-to-day activities. That is why I incorporate resistance exercises, both on gym equipment and with hand weights, into the program I present in this book.

Benefit 10: Fights Stress and Improves Mood

Worries, depression, and mood swings undermine your health, relationships, and work performance and reduce your sense of being in control. Research has shown that people who make exercise a regular part of their lifestyle experience stress reduction, improvement in moods, and a greater ability to handle the worries of daily life. Studies that compare the body chemistry of joggers and those who do resistance exercise with the body chemistry of sedentary individuals show a greater percentage of mood-elevating substances such as endorphins in the bloodstream of those who are regularly involved in some form of exercise.

One study on the psychological effects of exercise on people suffering from osteoarthritis showed that exercise

- Helped release pent-up feelings and improve mood
- Gave people a coping strategy for control of pain
- Increased levels of independence and feelings of self-sufficiency
- Increased self-esteem
- Improved social interaction

Kelly: Exercise Saved Me from Going Off the Deep End

Recently, I saw a remarkable example of how exercise works to combat stress. A former client named Kelly who'd had great success in my program told me a dramatic story of how exercise had literally saved her sanity during the most difficult six weeks of her life. "Mackie," she said, "you're not going to believe what's been happening with me. I think I'm going to have to change my name to Calamity Jane."

Kelly had been diagnosed with cancer a year earlier. She had a successful round of surgery and chemotherapy, but she was facing a final treatment consisting of six weeks of radiation therapy. Radiation is somewhat hard on the body because it lowers immune function, creates pain and swelling in the radiated area, and generally makes a person feel exhausted in the last three weeks of treatment. On top of this, she had to get up on Monday through Friday and drive to the treatment center, taking a big bite out of her workday.

Two weeks into her treatment, Kelly's grandmother died. Then during the last month of Kelly's treatment, her seventy-two-year-old mother was admitted to the hospital with dangerously high blood pressure and mental confusion. Her mom spent thirty days in the hospital. Because her mother lived 3,000 miles away and Kelly could not be with her, this was an agonizing experience. Since her sister had to bear the brunt of the hospital visits and medical decisions, Kelly felt completely stressed and helpless to do anything concrete for her family.

On top of everything else, Kelly was writing a book against a deadline. "Mackie," she told me, "if I hadn't been able to keep on exercising, I think I would have gone off the deep end. Luckily, I knew how to keep myself sane by keeping my body moving and by consciously managing my stress and eating right. What you taught me was a big factor in keeping myself together and moving forward with everything that I had to do without succumbing to overwhelming stress. I can't tell you how much better it made me feel to go to the gym or take a long, fast walk. No matter what, even if it meant walking back and forth on the pier by the ocean at eight o'clock at night in the dark, I always made time for exercise because I knew it was my lifeline."

Far too many North Americans don't exercise. And many of those who do often exercise without a real understanding of how to get the most out of their workout. They might go to the gym a few times a week, walk, bicycle, shoot some hoops, take an aerobics class now and again. While any kind of exercise benefits you and raises your overall level of health and well-being, the real issue is: How can you get the most out of each workout session?

Most people exercise with specific goals in mind: losing fat and inches, improving cardiovascular health, gaining more energy and peace of mind. But if you don't really know how to exercise effectively, you may never reach your goals. My Fat-Burning Metabolic Fitness Exercise Plan, a carefully structured combination of resistive training, cardio, a core body workout, and interval training, is designed to give you the best of all possible exercise worlds—and it only requires 300 minutes spread over six days a week, and even less as you progress beyond the basic four-week fat-loss program. No matter how out of shape and overweight you are, no matter how sluggish your metabolism, this program will transform your body into a fat-burning machine in as little as twenty-eight days.

This program represents what I have learned over my thirty-year career as a top performance enhancement expert. It is based on the following:

1. The very latest health- and sports-related research
2. My years of experience helping world-class athletes and others to achieve their highest levels of performance while teaching them how to expend their energy in the most efficient way possible
3. My years of experience designing programs to help overweight, obese, and morbidly obese men and women lose fat and regain their health

To help you to get the most out of this exercise program, let's take a look at how it is designed and why. There are detailed instructions in chapter 13 on how to perform all of the exercises, along with photographs and guidelines.

Learn How to Exercise at the Right Level of Intensity

One of the most significant factors in achieving maximum fat loss is learning how to exercise at the right intensity level. Most of us who belong to a gym are familiar with those who sweat and strenuously exercise until their veins look like they are about to pop. This intensity level may be dangerous. One client told me a story of a terribly overweight man who seemed to live at the gym. "No matter which morning I went in for my workout, there he was, straining to lift massive amounts of weight on every machine he used, apparently for a couple of hours each day. One day he just disappeared and I never saw him again. When I asked one of the trainers what had happened to him, he told me that the man had given himself a hernia. I felt sorry for him because he was trying so hard. But I could have predicted what happened because he didn't know how to work at a level of intensity that he could handle."

With any type of exercise, it is the quality of effort that counts rather than the quantity. Everyone has heard the expression "give it 100 percent." But the truth is that you can only give 100 percent for a very short period of time without becoming totally exhausted and compromising the effectiveness of your workout. The strongest effort that you can maintain consistently is closer to 80 percent of your maximum.

Our goal in this exercise program is not maximum effort but doing each type of exercise at a level of intensity, based on your gender, which will guarantee the greatest amount of fat loss and increased metabolic efficiency in the shortest amount of time. Because somewhat different hormonal responses occur during fat storage and fat metabolism in each gender, men and women tend to respond best to different exercise intensities. According to a study published by the IDEA Health and Fitness Source, women lose more fat by exercising at low to moderate levels of intensity while men seem to lose more fat by exercising at moderate to high levels of intensity. The reason is that women sustain a lower respiratory exchange rate (RER) than men during exercise at lower intensities. RER is the numeric index that indicates the amount of carbohydrates and fat used during exercise based on the ratio between the amount of carbon dioxide you produce in relationship to the amount of oxygen you consume. The lower the RER, the more fat being burned as fuel.

A recent article in the *International Journal of Sport Nutrition and Exercise* supports this finding further by reporting that women have a lower RER than men during prolonged exercise in a fasted state—in other words, before meals. While both genders will get the most out of their exercise if they do it on an empty stomach, this is especially so for women. If a woman eats some kind of carbohydrate, such as a power bar or a protein drink, before exercising, she will tend to use that as fuel. On an empty stomach, she will use greater amounts of internal fat and stored carbohydrates as a metabolic fuel source. This study also showed that women who are still menstruating are at their fat-burning height in the week following their cycle.

The Rate of Perceived Exertion: Instinctive Intensity Training

The simplest and most effective way to monitor your intensity level so that you get the most out of your workout is by using my Instinctive Intensity Training (IIT) Scale based on the rate of perceived exertion. Once you have checked with your doctor to make sure that there are no restrictions on your ability to exercise, go to your gym, warm up carefully, then see what you would consider to be your maximum effort. If you are overfat and are at risk (see the PAR-Q Questionnaire in chapter 13), you may choose to perform this maximum effort test as part of a pulmonary stress test in the presence of your physician or a cardiologist. Your insurance may pay for this test with the appropriate diagnosis and CPT code.

Once you've identified what your maximum effort feels like, use the following scale to find the appropriate IIT zone for your workout:

INSTINCTIVE INTENSITY TRAINING SCALE

IIT Level	Percentage of Maximum Effort	Perception
4	40	Warm-up effort
6	60	Mild effort
7	70	Moderate effort
8	80	Strong effort
9	90	Very strong effort
10	100	Maximum effort

The concept behind the IIT scale is that no one can tell you exactly how many pounds you need to use or how vigorously you need to exercise. How you perceive whether an exercise is low, moderate, or high intensity is a subjective experience based on your general level of fitness. A level of effort that seems easy for one person might present a challenge to another person, especially if he or she is deconditioned, is overweight, or hasn't exercised for a while.

To find your appropriate IIT level, you must learn to listen to your body. That means paying attention to a broad spectrum of physical sensations, including fatigue levels, muscle or leg pain, physical stress, and shortness of breath. For each type of exercise I am asking you to do, you need to estimate how hard you need to work to achieve the desired level of intensity.

Research has shown that your perception of the amount of effort you feel you are putting into an activity is likely to agree with the actual physical measurements of that effort—that is, if you feel you are exercising moderately, measurements of things such as how fast your heart is beating would probably confirm that you are exercising at a moderate level. For example, during moderate activity you can sense that you are challenging yourself but are not yet near your limit.

The cardiovascular and interval training exercises in my program are designed to be performed at a gender-specific intensity level that will enable you to achieve your metabolic and fat-burning goals.

13

The Fat-Burning Workout

Module 1, the basic program, consists of 4 weeks of exercise specifically designed to exponentially raise your fat-burning ability and metabolism to a much higher level. If you wish to take advantage of this newfound metabolic efficiency and continue further, I am offering you two additional 4-week programs, which I call Module 2 and Module 3. With each module, the amount of time spent exercising becomes shorter, but the intensity and number of repetitions increases. While you are spending 300 minutes exercising in Module 1, you are doing so at a low to moderate intensity level. By the time you reach Module 3, you are exercising for only 200 minutes per week, but at moderate to high intensities. I also provide a maintenance program that will help you to stay fit for life.

Module 1

Module 1 is a basic 4-week plan that can be used as a stand-alone rapid fat-loss program. I euphemistically call this 4-week program my "boot camp" because the results are so phenomenal. A client named Angela is a case in point. She lost 15 pounds, 6 percent body fat, and 4 inches from her waistline in only a single month.

Module 1, which is a total of 300 minutes of exercise per week, is set up as follows:

Module 1: Days 1, 3, and 5

Circuit Training. On days 1, 3, and 5 you will do 10 minutes a day of circuit training alternating between the upper and lower body. You can do this either in the gym (10 reps on 10 machines) or at home (10 reps of 10 resistance exercises, some using dumbbells). You will have 1 minute to complete each exercise, comprised of 20 seconds of active work, followed by 40 seconds of active rest (moving to the next machine and setting the pin for the next exercise).

Circuit or resistive training has several benefits. It is an anaerobic form of exercise, which means that it creates an oxygen debt—you get out of breath when you do it. When an oxygen debt is created, the body moves from burning fat to burning carbohydrates that are stored in the muscles, in the liver, and to a lesser degree in the circulatory system. Anaerobic resistance exercise increases your metabolism by maintaining your lean body mass (fat-free tissue), which is your metabolically active tissue. In this type of exercise, even after your session is complete, your metabolic rate is still at an active level for up to 48 hours.

The reason for this is a mechanism known as excess postexercise oxygen consumption (EPOC). People always knew that steady-state cardiovascular exercise burned fat. But based on my experience in helping professional boxers lose weight, I have found that circuit training can have the same effect.

The EPOC effect helps you lose tremendous amounts of weight but still stay strong because you are in a hypermetabolic state. The effect on the muscles caused by circuit training increases your ability to efficiently metabolize the foods you eat, especially carbohydrates. When you combine exercise training with a 25 percent balanced energy reduction in your diet, which is what we are doing in this program, you get a heightened metabolic rate.

A study published in the *International Journal of Sport Nutrition and Exercise,* structured along the exact same lines as my circuit training program, showed that a session of resistive exercise done at a moderate intensity, in a 2:1 ratio of work and active rest, increased metabolism for up to 48 hours.

Circuit training also has a positive effect on the hormones. The American College of Sports Medicine reports that when muscles contract and relax during multiple sets of resistive exercise, the body is stimulated to produce significant levels of human growth hormone and testosterone. When a critical level in the anaerobic threshold is passed, there is also a sharp rise in the hormone epinephrine, which stimulates the burning of fat.

Cardio Training. Each 10-minute session of circuit training in Module 1 will be followed by 50 minutes of cardio training. Whereas circuit training alternates between work and active rest, the cardio training is steady state. For this form of exercise, the intensity level for men should be 4.5 to 5 on the IIT scale. For women it should be 3.5 to 4.5. Remember, women should do their cardio at a lower rate because studies have shown that women burn greater amounts of fat at low to moderate intensities compared to men. It does not matter what kind of cardio you do—walking outside or on a treadmill, working out on a cross-trainer, bicycling, swimming; it just matters that you do it at the proper intensity and for the correct amount of time.

Because this exercise is steady state, this is the aerobic, or fat-burning, part of the program. Since the body's fat-burning capacity reaches its maximum after 20 minutes of cardio done at the proper level of intensity, 50 minutes gives you 30 minutes of almost pure fat loss. As you become more metabolically fit, you will begin to maximize fat loss earlier in your cardio session.

The importance of cardio training cannot be underestimated. A recent study published by the American College of Sports Medicine has shown that poor cardiovascular health is associated with an increased incidence of type 2 diabetes, heart disease, high cholesterol, and hypertension. It is also connected to the cluster of symptoms we call Metabolic Syndrome X. Men who had low levels of physical activity had a seven times greater chance of developing Metabolic Syndrome than men who engaged in moderate to high levels of cardiovascular exercise. Women are equally at risk.

An article in the *Medical Tribune* showed that the risk of developing heart disease decreased 15 percent for every half mile walked per day. By walking 2 miles per day, you can decrease your risk for coronary disease by over 50 percent.

A recent study published in *Medicine and Science in Sports & Exercise* reports that regular cardiovascular exercise done at the proper intensity has also been shown to decrease inflammatory markers in the blood. Inflammatory markers, such as C-reactive protein, contribute to the risk of cardiovascular disease.

Days 1, 3, and 5 of the program add up to 60 minutes total per day or 180 minutes per week of the 300 minutes total for Module 1. The primary goal of these three days is to preserve muscle mass (circuit training) and to burn fat (cardio).

Module 1: Days 2, 4, and 6

Core Exercises. On days 2, 4, and 6 in Module 1 you will be doing core (midbody/abdominal) exercises for 10 minutes a day. Each exercise will be comprised of 10 repetitions and the work-to-active rest ratio will be 1:2. You will be allowed a total of 1 minute for each exercise divided into 20 seconds of work and 40 seconds of active rest (time allowed to get into position for the next exercise).

Core exercises have several benefits. As a form of anaerobic exercise, they increase your metabolic rate. Core exercises also selectively work the abdominal area where fat represents the greatest risk to your health. Another benefit is that they improve glucose tolerance by enhancing insulin sensitivity of the beta receptors (see chapter 3 for a discussion of beta receptors).

Core exercises will not only melt inches off your waistline. They will also improve your performance in other types of exercise because they increase power and flexibility in the central part of your body. Most men and women who carry abdominal fat suffer from constant pain in their lower back due to structural instability. Core exercises will help you to develop a strong functional pelvic area and live without chronic backaches. If you are always visiting the chiropractor because your back keeps going out of alignment, these kinds of exercises will keep you stable for longer and longer periods of time. My chiropractor and many others stress the importance of doing these kinds of exercises.

Interval Training. On days 2, 4, and 6 you will also be doing 30 minutes of interval training. In Module 1, these exercises will be performed at a 1:2 ratio of work to active rest. In this case, your active rest will be comprised of a 10-minute warm-up, followed by 10 minutes of interval training, followed by a 10-minute cool-down.

The interval section of this exercise session will be divided into 10 discreet units of 1 minute each. Each minute is comprised of 20 seconds of high-intensity work where you are pushing yourself and 40 seconds of lower-intensity work.

Men should do the higher-intensity portion of their interval training at an IIT level of 6 to 9, women on a level of 6 to 8. Notice that I am asking you to push yourself relatively hard during this part of the interval training.

I also suggest that you don't just perform the higher-intensity part of this exercise at one level. Try to vary the intensity during each discreet unit of the active work phase. Women may be performing some intervals at 6, some at 7, and some at 8. I know this is a lot to concentrate on when you are trying to count off 20-second intervals of active work and 40-second intervals of active rest. But as you get more comfortable with interval training, you will be able to add this varying intensity element to your workout with ease.

For both men and women the active-rest phase of each minute of interval training should be performed at a level of 3 to 4 on the IIT scale. The warm-up and cool-down periods for both men and women should also be performed at IIT levels of 3 to 4.

Interval training can include fast walking, sprinting, bicycling, working on the cross-trainer, and so on, as long as you vary your intensity levels according to the plan. Interval training gives you the best of both worlds since it strengthens your body both anaerobically and aerobically. Like resistance exercise, it is anaerobic and will elevate your metabolism and enhance the thermic effect of food digestion for up to 48 hours. A recent study published at MuscleMedia.com reported that interval training caused greater fat loss than endurance training. The study group that exercised over time using short bursts of high-intensity interval training lost nine times as much fat as the study group that performed 45 minutes of high-intensity training. Levels of HGH, testosterone, and estrogen were also significantly higher after bouts of interval training as opposed to endurance training. Interval training is a type of exercise where less effort—short bursts of intensity—will get you much better results than long bouts of intense effort.

Core exercises for 10 minutes followed by interval training for 30 minutes comes out to 120 minutes (40 minutes × 3) per week of the 300 minutes total in Module 1. The primary goal of these three days is to increase metabolism by raising your anaerobic threshold.

In Module 1, the basic fat-loss program, the total minutes spent exercising per week add up to 300 minutes (a total of 180 minutes for days 1, 3, and 5 plus a total of 120 minutes for days 2, 4, and 6).

Why 300 Minutes?

When I ask you to exercise for 300 minutes a week, this is not an arbitrary number I picked out of the air. Dozens of studies have proven that one of the fundamental principles for successful fat loss and metabolic efficiency is exercising for the proper amount of time. The most recent data from the National Weight Control Registry show that a minimum of 225 minutes of moderate-intensity exercise per week results in a significant amount of fat loss. This study also shows that at least 225 minutes per week is an effective treatment modality for people suffering from Metabolic Syndrome X.

Since you expend roughly 100 calories for every 10 minutes spent exercising, 300 minutes will result in an approximate caloric expenditure of 3,000 calories per week during the first Module. I have found that this much exercise done over a 4-week period, coupled with the metabolic nutrition plan can result in a loss of as much as 14 pounds.

Some people may be satisfied with their results in Module 1. But if you wish to continue to reap greater benefits from your increased metabolism and capacity for fat loss, you may continue on with Modules 2 and 3, followed by my metabolic maintenance plan.

Module 2

Since your metabolism is now much more efficient than it was when you began, Module 2 cuts back from 6 days of exercise per week to 5 days.

Module 2: Days 1, 3, and 5

Circuit Training. Because you are now stronger and these exercises should be getting easier, in Module 2 you will increase your number of circuits from one to two. I also double your total time spent doing the entire routine from 10 minutes to 20 minutes to give you time to complete both circuits. Again, you will be working on a 1:2 ratio of 20 seconds of work to 40 seconds of active rest.

You will follow the same format in the at-home program, doubling the number of reps and the times in which you do them.

Cardio. Since you are now more metabolically efficient—more of a fat-burning machine—the amount of time you are doing your cardio can be reduced to 40 minutes of steady state. To get the same benefits from this time period as from the original 50-minute cardio session, I am asking you to increase your intensity. Men will now be doing their cardio at an IIT level of 5.5 to 7 and women at a level of 4.5 to 6.

Total time spent weekly on the circuit training and cardio will continue to be 60 minutes per day, for a total of 180 minutes of the 260 total per week in Module 2.

Module 2: Days 2 and 4

Core Exercises. Since you are now stronger and more metabolically efficient, I am asking you to do 15 repetitions of each exercise instead of 10. In this case, you will be doing those 15 reps within the same time period—20 seconds. So, your ratio of work to active rest will continue to be 1:2—20 seconds of work and 40 seconds to change to the next position. Your total time spent doing core exercises will continue to be 10 minutes.

Interval training. The total time spent doing the interval training session continues to be 30 minutes—10 minutes of warm-up, 10 minutes of 10 discreet intervals timed at 1 minute each, and 10 minutes of cool-down. The difference is that now I am asking you to restructure the intervals to 30 seconds of active work and 30 seconds of active rest (a 1:1 work-to-rest ratio). While the intensity level of the warm-up, active rest, and cool-down will continue to be 3 to 4 on the IIT scale for both men and women, I'm going to ask you to increase the level of your active work during each 1-minute interval to 7 to 9 on the IIT scale for men and 7 to 8 for women.

Core exercises for 10 minutes followed by interval training for 30 minutes done 2 days a week comes out to 80 minutes (40 × 2) of the 260 total per week.

In the second module, the total minutes spent exercising per week comes out to 260 minutes (a total of 180 minutes for days 1, 3, and 5 plus a total of 80 minutes for days 2 and 4), enabling significant fat loss, especially since you are now carrying less body fat and are more metabolically efficient.

Module 3

Since your metabolism is continuing to become more and more efficient with each passing month, Module 3 cuts back from 5 days of exercise per week to 4 days.

Module 3: Days 1 and 4

Circuit Training. Because you are getting stronger as the weeks pass and the exercises should be getting easier, in Module 3 I decrease your number of days to 2 per week but increase your workout to three circuits of 10 reps each. I also increase your total time spent doing this exercise routine from 20 minutes to 30 minutes to give you time to complete all three circuits. You will be working on a 1:2 ratio of 20 seconds of work to 40 seconds of active rest. You will follow the same format in the at-home circuit program.

Cardio. Since you are now more metabolically efficient, the amount of time you are doing your cardio can be reduced to 30 minutes of steady state. To get the same benefits from this time period as from the 40-minute time period in Module 2, I am asking you to increase your intensity. Men will be doing their cardio at an IIT level of 7 to 8 and women at a level of 6 to 7.

Total time spent weekly on the circuit training and cardio will continue to be 60 minutes per day, coming to a total of 120 minutes of the 200 minutes per week in Module 3.

Module 3: Days 2 and 5

Core Exercises. Since you are now stronger and more metabolically efficient, I am asking you to do 20 repetitions of each exercise instead of 15. You will continue to do those 20 reps within the same time period—20 seconds. Your ratio of work to active rest will continue to be 1:2—20 seconds of work and 40 seconds to change to the next position. Your total time spent doing core exercises will continue to be 10 minutes.

Interval Training. The total time spent for the interval training session continues to be 30 minutes—10 minutes of warm-up, 10 minutes of 10 discreet intervals of 1 minute each, and 10 minutes of cool-down. The difference is that I am now asking you to restructure the intervals to a ratio of 2:1, which comes out to 40 seconds of active work and 20 seconds of active rest. The intensity level of the warm-up, active rest, and cool-down will continue to be 3 to 4 on the IIT scale for both men and women. But since the length of the active work part of the interval has increased significantly, I'm going to allow you to decrease the level of your active work intensity down to 7 to 8 on the IIT scale for men and 6 to 7 for women.

Core exercises for 10 minutes followed by interval training for 30 minutes done 2 days a week comes out to 80 minutes (40 minutes × 2) per week.

In the third module, the total minutes spent exercising per week comes out to 200 minutes per week (120 minutes for days 1 and 3 plus 80 minutes for days 2 and 4).

The Fat-Burning Metabolic Fitness Maintenance Program

Once you have completed Modules 1, 2, and 3, you will be able to switch to my maintenance program, which simply involves 150 minutes of moderate-intensity exercise at an IIT level of 7 to 8 for men and 6 to 7 for women. All that is required for this part of the program is that you perform two circuit/resistive training sessions coupled with two sessions of steady-state cardio, and two interval training sessions coupled with two sessions of the core exercise routine. You may designate the number of minutes you spend doing these exercises in any way you see fit as long as your total time spent exercising comes out to 150 minutes.

Consult with Your Doctor before You Begin

Before beginning any exercise program, it is important that you consult with your doctor, especially if you have not exercised in a while and know or suspect that you have significant health problems. If you have taken the self-evaluation health tests in chapters 2, 4, 5, 6, and 7, you should have a fairly good idea of the state of your general health. Another important screening tool is the Physical Activity Readiness Questionnaire, more commonly known as the PAR-Q. This basic self-evaluation, developed by the Canadian Society for Exercise Physiology, has been clinically tested and shown to be an effective and reliable screening tool. Please answer these seven questions honestly.

PAR-Q and You
A Questionnaire for People Ages 15–69

Regular physical activity is fun and healthy, and increasingly more people are starting to become more active every day. Being more active is safe for most people. However, some people should check with their doctor before they start becoming much more physically active.

If you are planning to become more physically active than you are now, start by answering the seven questions below. If you are between the ages of fifteen and sixty-nine, the PAR-Q will tell you if you should check with your doctor before you start. If you are over sixty-nine years of age, and you are not used to being very active, check with your doctor.

Common sense is your best guide when you answer these questions. Please read the questions carefully and answer each one honestly yes or no.

	Yes	No
1. Has your doctor ever said that you have a heart condition *and* that you should only do physical activity recommended by a doctor?	☐	☐
2. Do you feel pain in your chest when you do physical activity?	☐	☐
3. In the past month, have you had chest pain when you were not doing physical activity?	☐	☐
4. Do you lose your balance because of dizziness or do you ever lose consciousness?	☐	☐
5. Do you have a bone or joint problem that could be made worse by a change in your physical activity?	☐	☐
6. Is your doctor currently prescribing drugs (for example, water pills) for your blood pressure or heart condition?	☐	☐
7. Do you know of any *other reason* why you should not do physical activity?	☐	☐

If you answered yes to one or more questions, you should talk with your doctor by phone or in person before you start becoming more physically active or before you have a physical appraisal. Tell your doctor about the PAR-Q and which questions you answered yes.

- You may be able to do any activity you want—as long as you start slowly and build up gradually. Or you may need to restrict your activities to those that are safe for you. Talk with your doctor about the kinds of activities in which you wish to participate and follow his/her advice.
- Find out which community programs are safe and helpful for you.

If you honestly answered no to all *PAR-Q questions,* you can be reasonably sure that you can:

- Start becoming more physically active—begin slowly and build up gradually. This is the safest and easiest way to go.
- Take part in a fitness appraisal—this is an excellent way to determine your basic fitness so that you can plan the best way for you to

live actively. It is also highly recommended that you have your blood pressure evaluated. If your reading is over 144/94, talk with your doctor before you start becoming more physically active.

Delay becoming much more active:

- If you are not feeling well because of a temporary illness such as a cold or a fever—wait until you feel better; or
- If you are or may be pregnant—talk to your doctor before you start becoming more active.

Note: If your health changes so that you then answer yes to any of the above questions, tell your fitness or health professional. Ask whether you should change your physical activity plan.

Informed use of the PAR-Q: The Canadian Society for Exercise Physiology, Health Canada, and their agents assume no liability for persons who undertake physical activity. If in doubt after completing the questionnaire, consult your doctor prior to physical activity.

Now that you have learned the basics about exercising safely and getting the most from your exercise regimen, let's move on to the exercises themselves.

The Workout

As you begin your first Fat-Burning Metabolic Fitness Exercise Plan workout, there are nine basic guidelines you should keep in mind.

1. *Orient yourself with the equipment.* One of the first things you should do before you begin is thoroughly familiarize yourself with the selectorized weight-training machines that you plan to use in your gym or the dumbbell routine that you will use at home. One of the gym's trainers can show you how to properly position your body for each exercise and can demonstrate appropriate lifting and breathing techniques for both the machines and the dumbbells. He or she can also help you select the proper starting weight for each machine.
2. *Always warm up your muscles first* with 5 or 10 minutes of light calisthenics or stretching exercise involving all parts of your body.

Spending 5 or 10 minutes on the treadmill to elevate your heart rate is also important.

3. *Move from exercise to exercise in the time of active rest allotted.* When you are doing the circuit part of the program, don't take more time than you are allowed to get yourself set up on the next machine. If you need to, practice adjusting the equipment seat and weights beforehand so that you can easily adjust the machine to your own specifications within the 40-second window of active rest. If a machine is in use by another gym patron, just move on to any type of machine that is free, as long as it is listed on the circuit workout and involves the proper part of the body—either upper body or lower body.

   When you are doing the core exercise sequence, practice the exercise positions beforehand so that you are familiar with them and don't have to waste a lot of time pondering over the book during your exercise session.

4. *Lift moderate weights.* When you are using a machine, lift only the amount of weight you can comfortably lift 10 times within 20 seconds. The correct amount of weight will be enough to make you feel as if you have reached the point of muscle fatigue by the end of your required reps. If it's too much weight, you won't be able to complete the set. If it's too little weight, you won't feel muscle tiredness at the end of your reps. Each lifting stroke should be relatively fast, with a well-controlled return. If you are not sure how much weight you should be lifting, ask a trainer. Don't risk injuring yourself. The same is true if you are doing your circuit training at home using free weights.

   While you will attempt to increase your weight by approximately 5 pounds each week to keep your body changing, never compromise your form, stability, alignment, or posture to increase the number of pounds you are lifting. The result is almost certain to be injury and poor posture. The best way to build strength is to maintain proper position and form during your workout, even if you are using only a relatively light amount of weight. Play it safe and never try to handle more weight than your body can stabilize.

5. *Maintain correct body positioning.* The most efficient position for the body while doing resistance training is one in which the spine is in a neutral position with a slight degree of straightening in the thoracic region (upper chest). This is accomplished by positioning

yourself comfortably against the backrest of the machine, then pushing your shoulders back slightly (known as scapular retraction) and lifting your chest slightly up and out. Positioning the spine in this manner is more efficient for supporting weight while still allowing for the least amount of intervertebral disk compression in the cervical (neck) and lumbar (lower back) regions. Also contract your abdominal muscles during lifting to help stabilize the lumbar spine.

When doing the core body exercises, make sure your back is supported by the floor and your limbs are aligned correctly. Avoid strain. Never force yourself beyond a range of motion that feels comfortable to you.

6. *Don't forget to breathe.* Keeping respiration going will keep your blood pressure from rising. Depending on the exercise, inhale when you extend and exhale on the way back in; inhale on the way down and exhale on the way out.

7. *Complete all repetitions.* If you are doing circuit exercises and the amount of weight you are using becomes heavy, stop the set, reduce the weight, and continue until you have completed the set of repetitions.

8. *Stay hydrated.* Make sure that you carry a bottle of water with you when exercising and take frequent drinks. You will want to drink between one-half and one entire 1.5-liter bottle of water per hour of workout time.

9. *Always cool down.* Finish your workout with a cool-down to decrease your pulse and breathing rates. Gradually reduce the intensity level until your pulse returns to a normal resting state. Then perform some easy, static stretching exercises to loosen tight muscles and increase flexibility.

Module 1: The Basic Four-Week Fat-Burning Program

Here is my basic Fat-Burning Metabolic Fitness Plan, which can be used as a stand-alone fat-loss workout. If you like the results you achieve at the end of four weeks and wish to take advantage of your heightened metabolism and fat-burning abilities to lose still more weight and inches, you may wish to continue on to Modules 2, 3, and the maintenance program.

At the end of four weeks, reevaluate your progress—inches lost, weight, body fat and lean muscle percentages, BMI, waist-to-hip ratio—using the charts in chapter 4.

Module 1: Days 1, 3, and 5

On any given day, you should do either the gym program or the home dumbbell program. You are not required to do both. For those who do not belong to a gym, the dumbbell program will be the only option. But either workout will give you the benefits of circuit training and will work the same muscle groups.

Gym Circuit Program

Frequency: 3 times per week

1 set of 10 reps for 10 exercises

A work/active rest ratio of 1:2 (20 seconds work, 40 seconds active rest)

Total circuit time: 10 minutes

Estimated calories expended: 100

Following are pictures of the ten exercises in the gym circuit program. The pictures illustrate correct positioning and are accompanied by descriptions of how to do each one correctly.

CHEST PRESS

1. Sit on the bench with your feet flat on the floor and slightly wider than shoulder width apart.
2. Grasp the handles and push outward until your arms are extended.
3. Return to the starting position and repeat for the required reps.

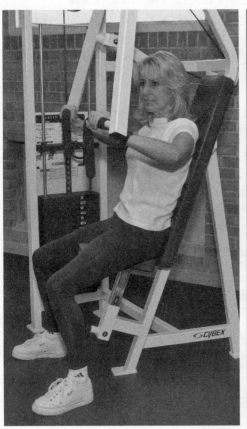 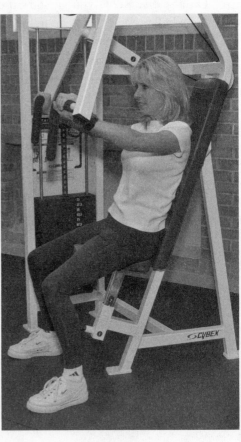

LEG PRESS

1. Sit on the bench so that your knees are at an angle of no more than 90 degrees. Grasp the handles for support.
2. Push on the platform with your feet until your legs are extended, keeping your knees slightly bent. Do not overextend.
3. Return to the starting position and repeat for the required reps.

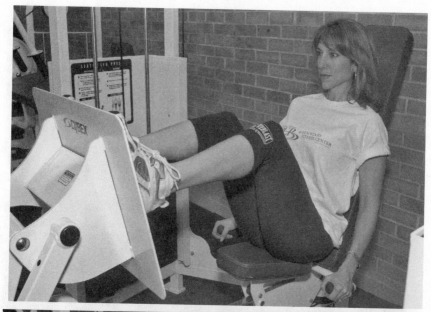

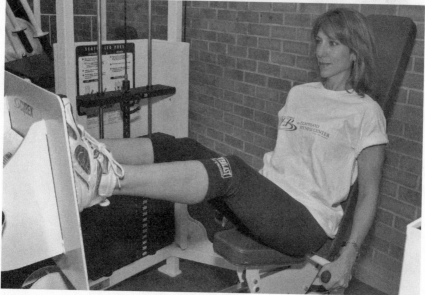

Seated Row

1. Sit on the bench with your feet flat on the floor and slightly wider than shoulder width apart. Your arms should be extended.
2. Grasp the handles with your palms facing down and pull back on the bars until your arms are bent at a 90-degree angle at the elbow. Do not let your elbows go past this point.
3. Return to the starting position and repeat for the required reps.

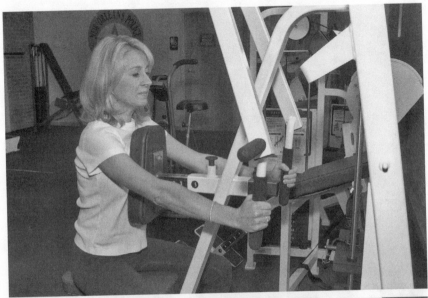

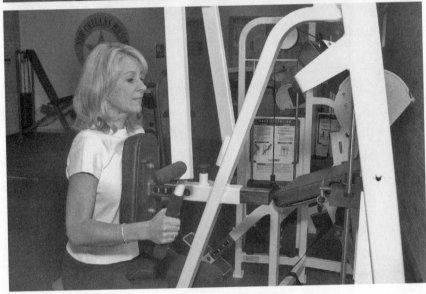

Leg Curl

1. Lie on your stomach on the bench. Grasp the handles provided for support. Place your legs under the bar at the ankle.
2. Curl your legs upward until your knees are at a 90-degree angle. Do not go past 90 degrees.
3. Return to the starting position and repeat for the required reps.

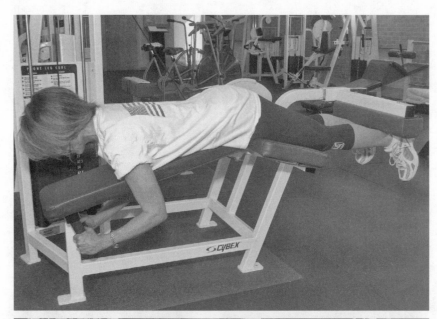

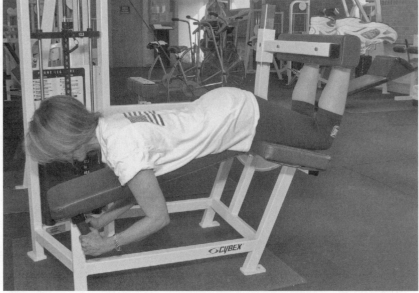

LATERAL PULL-DOWN

1. Sit at the machine with the bar above your thighs for support. Grasp the handles overhead with your palms facing in.
2. Pull down on the handles until they are close to your chest.
3. Return to the starting position and repeat for the required reps.

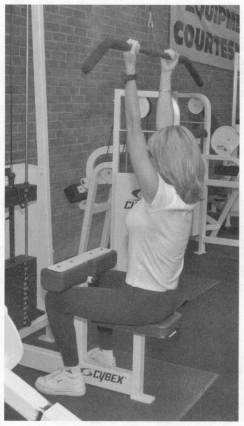
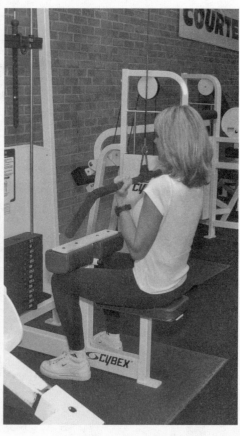

HIP ADDUCTION

1. Rotate machine roller so that it is 90 degrees from the floor (or at a comfortable height if you cannot lift your leg 90 degrees outward).
2. Stand comfortably with your hands on the machine handlebars and your feet together.
3. Keeping your knee slightly bent, lift your left leg and place it over the padded roller so that the roller is touching just below the knee. This might mean shifting the position of the standing leg. Do not lift your leg higher than 90 degrees.
4. While keeping the body straight and the hips aligned, contract the abdominals and push the padded roller downward toward the line of the body.
5. Return to the starting position and repeat for the required reps.
6. Repeat the entire exercise on the opposite side.

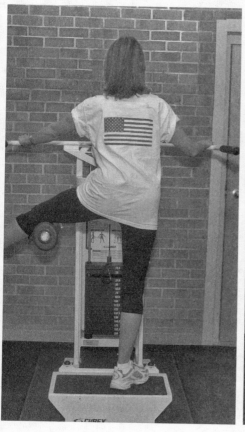
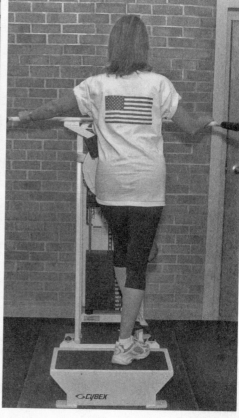

SHOULDER PRESS

1. Assume a comfortable position with your spine stabilized against the rear pad of the machine. Adjust the height of the seat so that your arms form a 90-degree angle at the elbow. In order to prevent an impingement of the shoulder joint, I recommend that you position your arms so that your palms face each other.
2. Elevate the bar to the full extension of your arms, keeping your elbows in during the movement. Exhale as you achieve the full extension of your arms.
3. Inhale on the return and repeat for the prescribed number of repetitions.

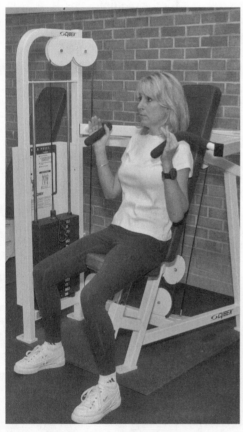 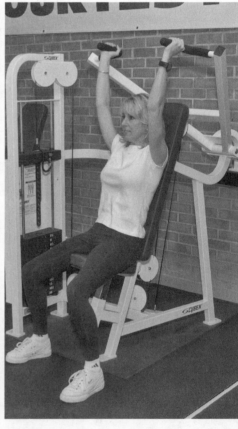

HIP ABDUCTION

1. Rotate the machine roller so that it is at its lowest position perpendicular to the floor.
2. Stand comfortably with your hands on the machine handlebars and your feet together.
3. Place the outside of your right thigh against the padded roller just above the knee.
4. While keeping the body straight and the hips aligned, contract the abdominals and lift the padded roller away from the body as high as you comfortably can.
5. Return to the starting position and repeat for the required reps.
6. Repeat the entire exercise on the opposite side.

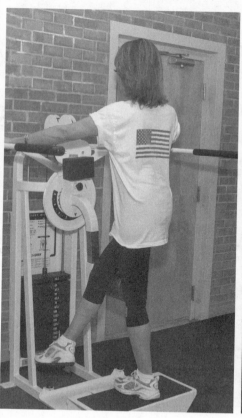
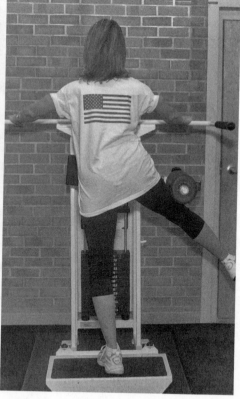

ABDOMINAL CRUNCH

1. Sit on the machine with your feet flat on the floor. Bend your arms at the elbows and rest them on the padded bar of the machine as shown.
2. In a slow and controlled manner, lean forward, pushing down on the bar. Use your abdominal muscles, not your arms, to control this motion. Hold for 3 to 5 seconds.
3. Return to the starting position and repeat for the required reps.

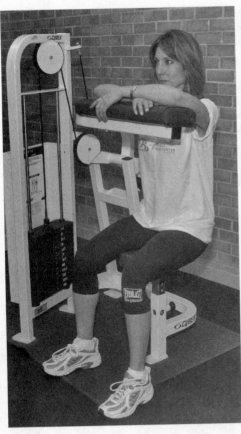 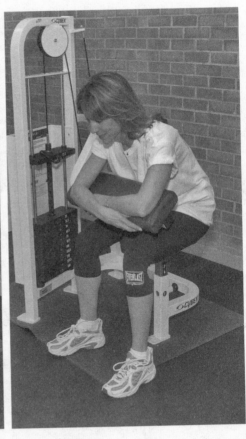

BACK EXTENSION

1. Sit on the bench with your feet solidly on the platform. Cross your arms in front of your chest. The pad should be resting just below your shoulders on your upper back.
2. Push against the pad to extend your back to a prone position. Do not overextend.
3. Return to the starting position and repeat for the required reps.

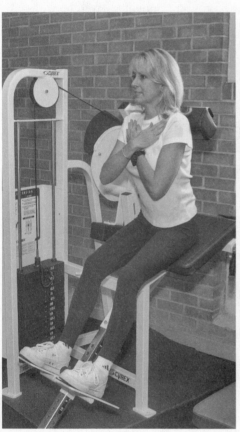 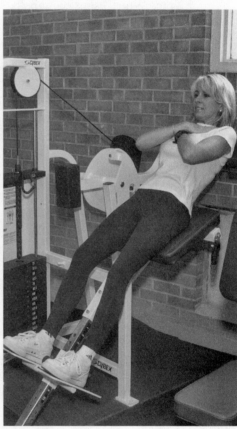

At-Home Circuit Program

Frequency: 3 times per week

1 set of 10 reps for 10 exercises

A work/active rest ratio of 1:2 (20 seconds work, 40 seconds active rest)

Total circuit time: 10 minutes

Estimated calories expended: 100

Note: When using dumbbells, use only an amount of weight with which you are comfortable. I suggest not exceeding 10 pounds for any exercise. You can buy dumbbells as light as 1 pound at sporting goods stores.

Following are pictures of the ten exercises in the at-home circuit program. The pictures illustrate correct positioning and are accompanied by descriptions of how to do each one correctly.

Push-up

1. Begin in position as shown.
2. Keeping your knees bent, push your chest away from the floor. Do not lock elbows at the end of the movement, but keep them slightly bent. Do not arch your back, but maintain a neutral neck and trunk alignment during the exercise.
3. Lower your body back down to the starting position and repeat for the required reps.

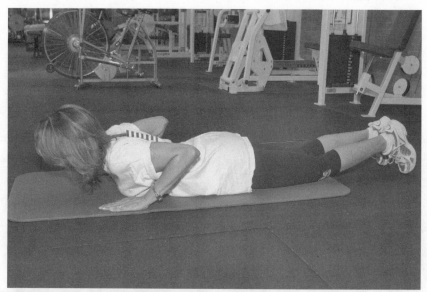

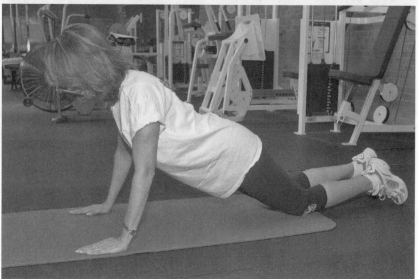

Wall Squat (may be done while holding dumbbells at your side)

1. Stand with your back against the wall (or an exercise ball—see photo) and your feet shoulder width apart.
2. Keeping your trunk stable by pressing your lower back gently into the wall or the exercise ball, lower your thighs until they are parallel with the floor. Do not let your hips drop below your knees. Try to keep your knees aligned over your feet during the exercise.
3. Return to the starting position and repeat for the required reps.

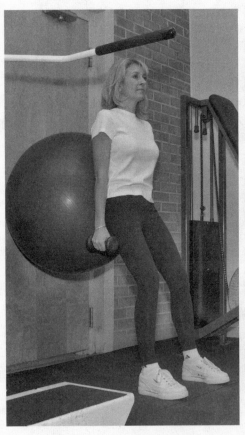 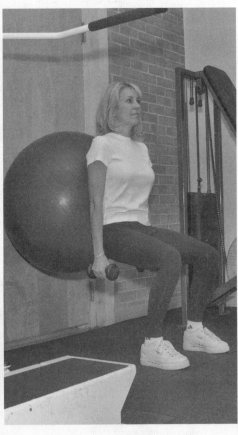

BENT-OVER ROW (HOLD DUMBBELL IN ACTIVE HAND)

1. Lean forward while resting one hand against a solid object such as a chair or a countertop, letting the other arm hang free.
2. Raise your unsupported arm backward and parallel with the chest while contracting your shoulder blade on that side. Do not allow your elbow to be raised above your back.
3. Slowly lower your arm to the starting position and repeat for the required reps.

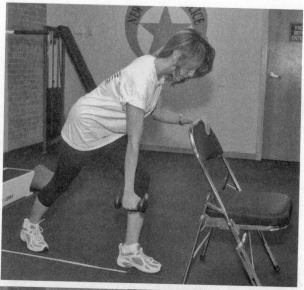

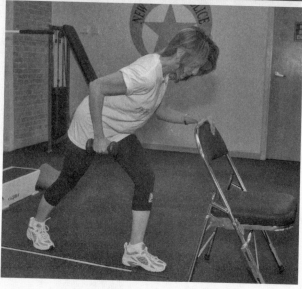

LUNGE (HOLD DUMBBELLS IN BOTH HANDS AT YOUR SIDES)

1. Stand with your feet together. Keeping your abdominals tight and your trunk upright, take a lunging step forward with one leg, as illustrated.
2. Lower your body until your thigh is nearly parallel to the floor. Keep your knee aligned with your foot, but do not allow it to extend over the front of your toes. If you experience any pain, modify the position of the lunge to be less deep.
3. Bring your leg back to the starting position and repeat with the opposite leg. Continue for the required reps.

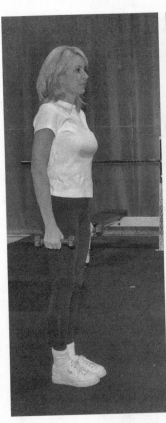
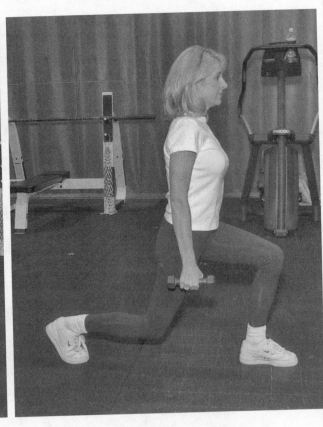

SHOULDER PRESS (PERFORM WITH DUMBBELLS)

1. Begin in a seated position with your elbows bent and positioned at your sides, as illustrated.
2. Keeping your palms facing inward and your thumbs stable, lift your arms overhead by extending your elbows. Do not lock your elbows at any time. If pain occurs in your shoulders, modify or stop the exercise.
3. Return to the starting position and repeat for the required reps.

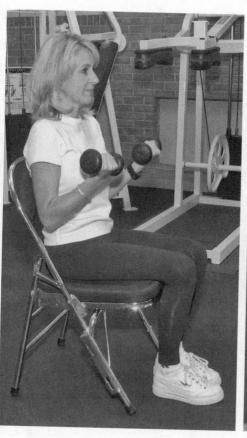 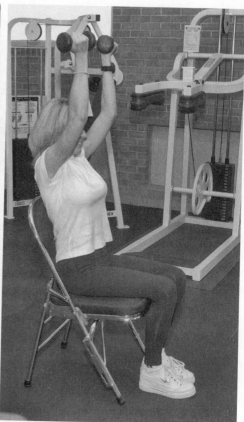

OUTER THIGH (USE A CUFF WEIGHT—A VELCRO WEIGHT THAT WILL ENCIRCLE YOUR ANKLE)

1. Lie on your side with your head resting in a neutral position on a 6–8-inch pillow when compressed (a folded towel is another option) and your hips stacked vertically. Bend your lower leg slightly.

2. Tighten your abdominals and lift your free leg, keeping it aligned with the trunk of your body and keeping your knee facing forward. Either lift it to the height shown in the picture or lower, as tolerated.

3. Return to the starting position. Repeat on the opposite side with the opposite leg. Continue for the required reps.

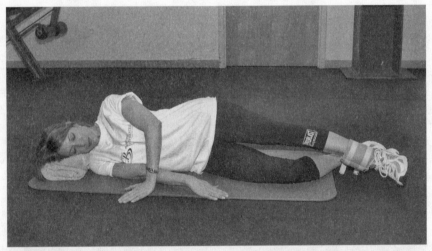

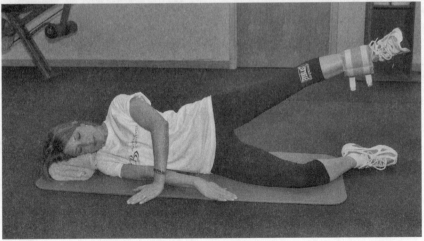

LATERAL RAISE (USE DUMBBELLS)

1. Stand with your knees slightly bent, your trunk stable, and your arms relaxed.
2. Raise your arms out to the sides with your thumbs pointing upward, stopping slightly below shoulder level. Do not lock your elbows.
3. Slowly return to the starting position and repeat for the required reps.

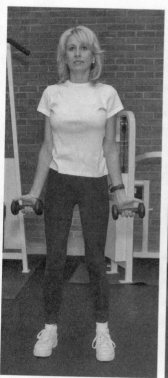 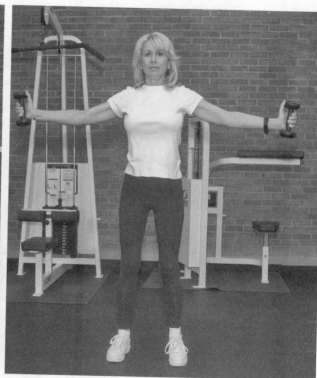

INNER THIGH (USE CUFF WEIGHT ON ANKLE)

1. Lie on your side propped up on your elbow with a folded towel or a 6–8–inch pillow under your elbow for comfort. Bend the knee of your top leg comfortably as shown.
2. Keeping your hips stacked vertically and your trunk stabilized, lift your bottom leg straight upward as shown in the picture or to a lower height as tolerated. Keep your knee facing straight ahead.
3. Return slowly to the starting position and repeat for the required reps.
4. Repeat the entire exercise on the opposite side.

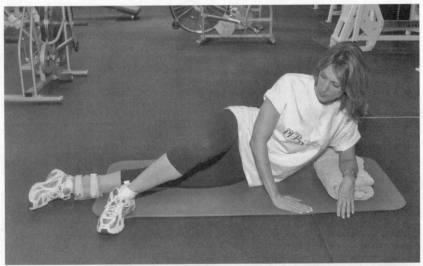

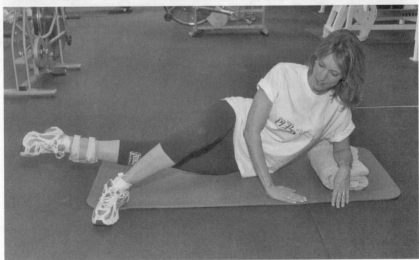

Standard Crunch (Upper Abdominals)

1. Lie on your back with your head on the floor and your arms crossed over your chest, legs bent and feet flat on the floor.
2. Raise your head and shoulders off the ground. Hold for a few seconds, then lower your head and shoulders to the starting position.
3. Repeat for the required reps.

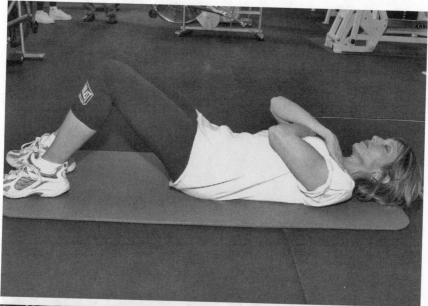

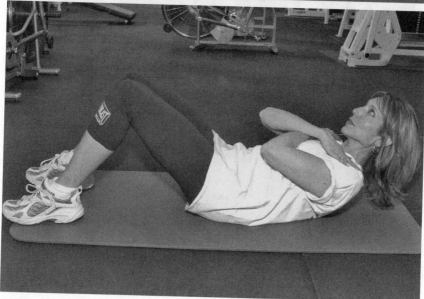

PRESS-UPS

1. Lie on your stomach in the position as shown.
2. Lift your chest upward as tolerated, keeping your hips pressed into the floor. Stop lifting if back pain or discomfort occurs.
3. Return to the starting position and repeat for the required reps.

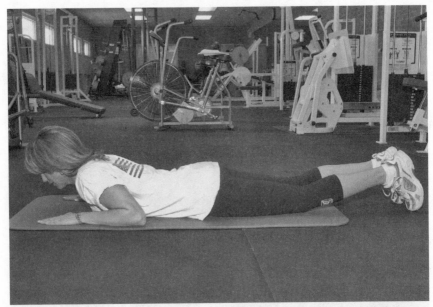

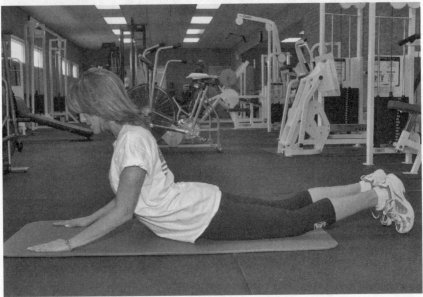

Module 1: Days 2, 4, and 6

Core Exercises

Frequency: 3 times per week

1 set of 10 reps for 10 exercises

A work/active rest ratio of 1:2 (20 seconds work, 40 seconds active rest)

Total time: 10 minutes

Estimated calories expended: 100

Following are pictures of the ten core exercises. The pictures illustrate correct positioning and are accompanied by descriptions of how to do each one correctly.

STANDARD CRUNCH (UPPER ABDOMINALS)

1. Lie on your back with your head on the floor and your arms crossed over your chest, legs bent and feet flat on the floor.
2. Raise your head and shoulders off the ground. Hold for a few seconds, then lower your head and shoulders to the starting position.
3. Repeat for the required reps.

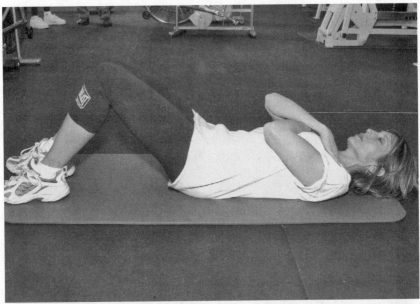

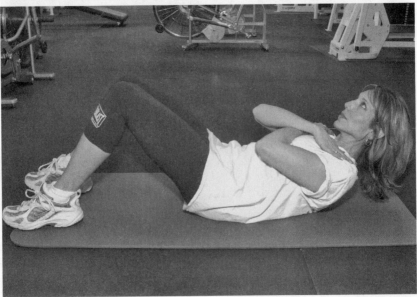

REVERSE CRUNCH (LOWER ABDOMINALS)

1. Lie on your back with your head on the floor, arms braced at your sides with palms on the floor. Legs are raised and knees bent at a right angle with calves parallel to the floor.
2. Begin by bringing your legs back toward your chest while contracting your lower abs. Slowly move back to the starting position.
3. Repeat for the required reps.

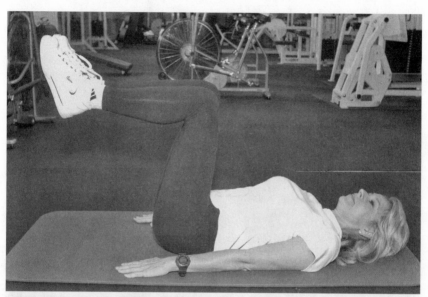

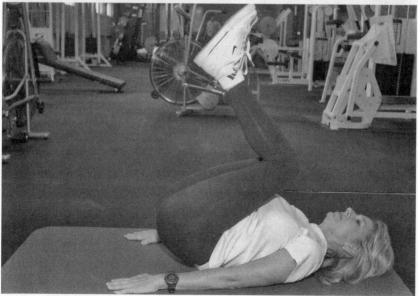

OBLIQUE CRUNCH

1. Lie flat on your back with your left foot flat on the floor. Cross the ankle of your right foot over your lower thigh.
2. Place your left hand to the side of your head, elbow out, and extend your other arm perpendicular to your side, palm down. Begin by curling your upper body forward at the waist.
3. Contract your torso across your midsection and try to touch your elbow to your knee (as shown). Squeeze your elbow to your knees.
4. Lower your body to the floor.
5. Switch legs and arms and repeat. Continue for the required reps.

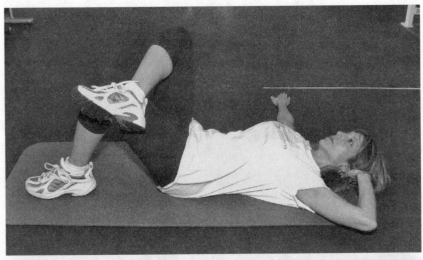

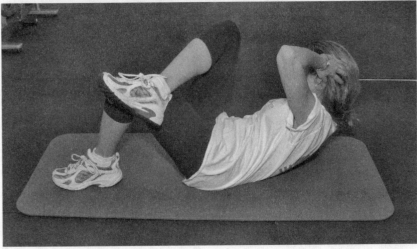

REVERSE TRUNK TWIST

1. Lie face up on the floor with your right arm out to the side, palm down, and your left arm bent with your hand behind your head.
2. Bend your knees.
3. While keeping your left foot flat on the floor, lift your right foot and rest your right ankle on top of your left knee as shown in the picture.
4. Keeping your right arm flat on the floor, contract your abs while lifting your head, right arm, and shoulder as shown in the picture. Inhale as you lift, and let your abs do the work of lifting, not your arm.
5. Using your abs, slowly lower your head, arm, and shoulder back down to the floor while exhaling. Repeat for the required number of reps.
6. Repeat the entire exercise on the opposite side.

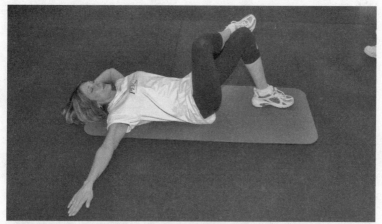

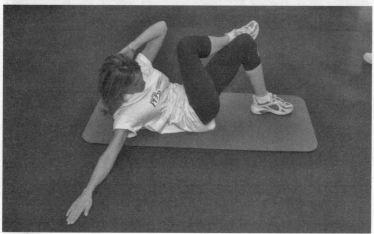

BRIDGE

1. Lie face up on the floor with your arms by your side, palms down, feet flat on the floor with your knees bent.
2. Tighten your abs and raise your trunk until your body forms a straight line between your knees and your shoulders.
3. Slowly lower yourself to the starting position and repeat for the required reps.

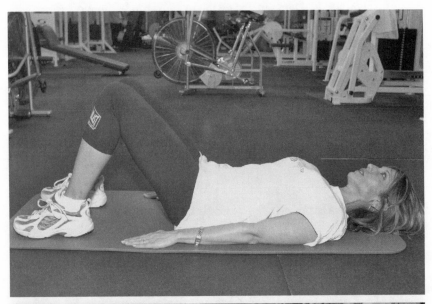

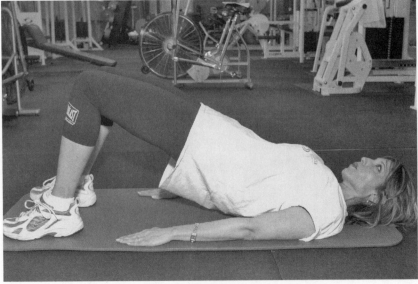

SUPERMAN OR SUPERWOMAN

1. Lie facedown on the floor with a 6–8–inch pillow when compressed (a folded towel is another option) under your lower abdominal pelvic region.
2. Raise your trunk, arms, and legs all at the same time so that your entire body is horizontal with the floor. Hold 2–3 seconds and relax.
3. Repeat for the required reps.
4. For a greater stretch, lift your trunk, arms, and left leg (high) while keeping your right leg on the floor. Hold 2–3 seconds and relax.
5. Repeat for the required number of reps.
6. Repeat the exercise lifting the opposite leg.

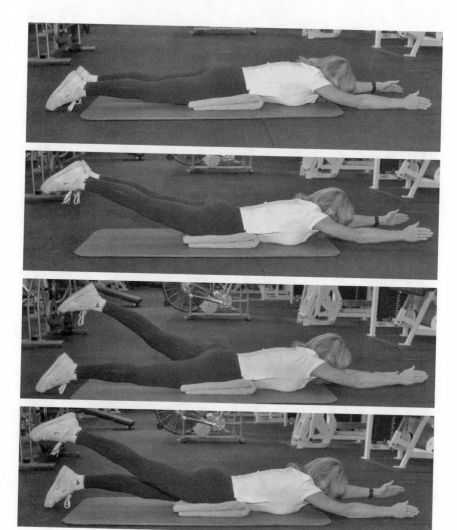

CROSS-BODY LIFT

1. Get down on all fours with your back straight.
2. Tighten your abdominal muscles and slowly raise one arm and its opposite leg until they are in line or slightly above the level of your back.
3. Slowly return to the starting position and repeat on the opposite side. Continue for the required reps.

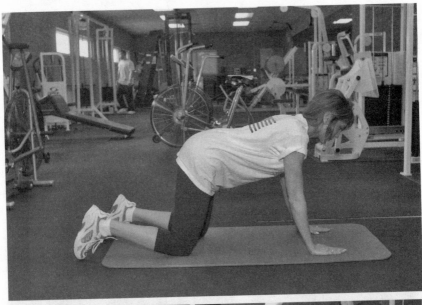

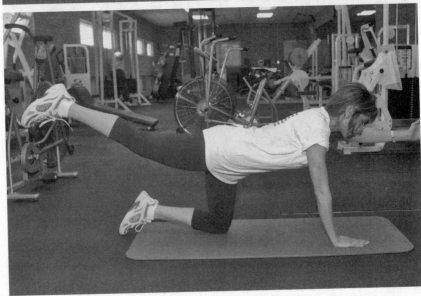

Back Raises

1. Lie facing the floor with your legs together and your upper body slightly raised and supported on your forearms.
2. Tighten your abs and raise your upper torso as far as you can without discomfort. Pause and flex the abdominal muscles for a few seconds, then lower yourself to the starting position.
3. Repeat for the required reps.

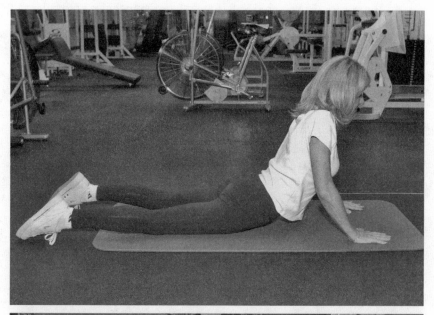

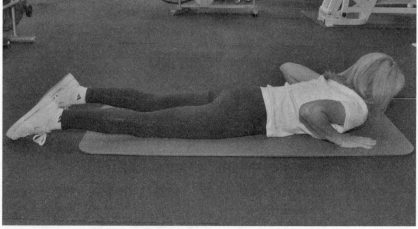

SIDE TWIST

1. Lie on the floor on your back with your hands behind your head, feet flat on the floor, and knees bent.
2. Keeping your shoulders on the floor, drop your knees to the right and touch them to the floor. Pause and flex your abdominal muscles for a few seconds.
3. In one continuous motion, raise your knees and drop them to the left. Exhale as you lower your legs and inhale as you raise them.
4. Repeat for the required reps. One repetition includes both sides.

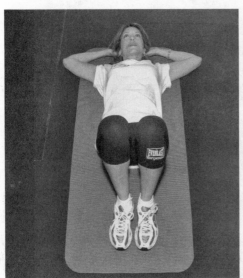 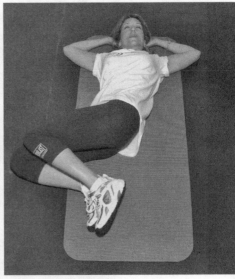

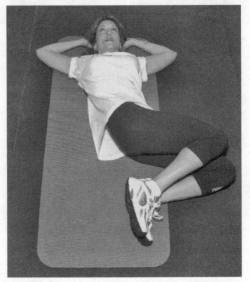

Cat Stretch

1. Get down on all fours with your back straight and your hands and knees shoulder width apart.
2. Begin by inhaling, then exhale as you pull your stomach to your spine, rounding your back upward and dropping your head until you are looking toward your pelvis. Feel this movement in your lower back.
3. Lower your back, inhale as you pass through the neutral position, then exhale as you bring your head up, pulling your shoulders down as you feel your spine extend.
4. Repeat in each direction three times.

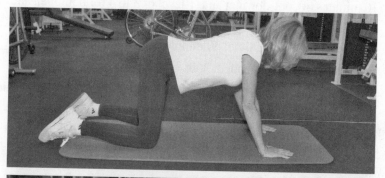

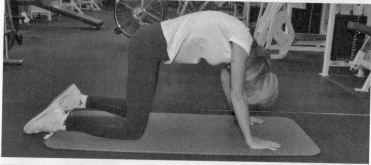

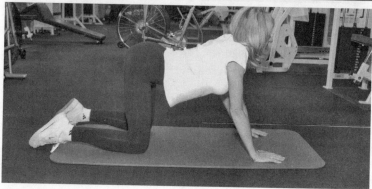

Interval Training

Frequency: 3 times per week

10 minutes of warm-up at an IIT level of 3 to 4 for both men and women

10 sets of intervals, each one lasting 1 minute

A work/active rest ratio of 1:2

20 seconds work at a higher intensity: 6 to 9 for men and 6 to 8 for women

40 seconds of work at a lower intensity: 3 to 4 for both men and women

10 minutes of cool-down at an IIT level of 3 to 4 for both men and women

Total interval training time: 30 minutes

Estimated calories expended: 300

You may do the exercise of your choice—walking or jogging outside, cross-trainer, treadmill, bicycling, jumping rope, and so on—as long as you adhere to the interval format of the program. Note: Remember to vary the intensity of your active work phase within each discreet interval. For example, if you are a man, do some intervals at 6, some at 7, some at 8, and some at 9 on the IIT scale.

Modules 2 and 3

To keep your body changing and yourself interested, you might wish to change the order of the exercises for Modules 2 and 3. I have suggested a format for you.

MODULE 2: SUGGESTED ORDER OF EXERCISES

Gym Circuit	*At-Home Circuit*	*Core Exercises*
Shoulder Press	Shoulder Press	Cat Stretch
Leg Curl	Lunge	Side Twist
Lateral Pull-down	Bent-over Row	Back Raises
Leg Press	Wall Squat	Cross-Body Lift
Seated Row	Push-up	Superman or Superwoman
Hip Abduction	Inner Thigh	Bridge
Chest Press	Lateral Raise	Reverse Trunk Twist
Hip Adduction	Press-ups	Oblique Crunch

| Back Extension | Standard Crunch | Reverse Crunch |
| Abdominal Crunch | Leg Curl | Standard Crunch |

MODULE 3: SUGGESTED ORDER OF EXERCISES

Gym Circuit	*At-Home Circuit*	*Core Exercises*
Leg Press	Lunge	Superman or Superwoman
Shoulder Press	Push-ups	Cross-Body Lift
Leg Curl	Wall Squat	Back Raises
Chest Press	Push-ups	Side Twist
Hip Abduction	Inner Thigh	Cat Stretch
Lateral Pull-down	Lateral Raise	Bridge
Hip Adduction	Outer Thigh	Reverse Trunk Twist
Seated Row	Bent-over Row	Oblique Crunch
Abdominal Crunch	Standard Crunch	Reverse Crunch
Back Extension	Press-ups	Standard Crunch

The Fat Dropped Off Like Crazy

An established boxer came to my program because he was getting ready to challenge for the Junior Welter Weight title. In order to qualify for the fight, he had to get his weight down from 175 to 140 pounds within three months. The challenge was that he could not afford to lose this fat at the expense of strength and stamina. He could not, as he had done in the past, skip meals to lose the weight. This was one of the most important fights of his career and there was too much at stake.

I designed a workout for him very similar to the one described in this chapter. I stressed that while I was pushing him to increase his metabolism, he had to support this level of exercise with balanced nutrition. I have found that most people who are overfat are usually doing what this young boxer did—skipping meals and overeating at the one or two meals a day that they allow themselves.

At first this seemed like a strange concept to him—working out harder and eating more often. But as the synergy of a metabolic exercise program and the balanced energy (caloric) deficit of my nutritional program went into effect, his body began to burn fat so efficiently that he lost 14 pounds in four weeks!

His energy levels went up as well. In the past, he usually felt drained during the months when he was getting ready for a fight. This time around, he's feeling better and stronger than he's ever felt. "I've never seen anything like this because I'm eating three meals a day and dropping weight like crazy, and my competition is probably starving himself." In his case, this program is definitely the prescription he needs, because on the night of the big fight he's going to be facing an opponent who will not have the metabolic fire and focus that he now has.

PART FOUR

The Four-Week Fat-Burning Plan

14

Map Your Progress:
Your Daily Fat-Burning
Metabolic Fitness
Evaluation Guide

Before you begin mapping your progress on my four-week program, I'd like to give you a tool called a Wellness Organizer that I offer each of my clients when they join my Fat-Burning Metabolic Fitness Plan. It gives you some basic tips to help maximize your fat loss.

The Fat-Burning Wellness Organizer

This system is a variation on the "Skinny Box" initially developed by Hal C. Becker, PhD, my field faculty advisor in graduate school. This Wellness Organizer has twelve categories designed to enhance your overall wellness profile. The thousands of clients I have worked with have shown that if a person uses the Wellness Organizer to its fullest extent, he or she will lose a minimum of 2 pounds of fat per week. The behavioral modification categories included in the wellness organizer are as follows:

Category 1: Calories in the kitchen. Place all food in the kitchen. Eating only in a designated area such as the kitchen or dining room will help you to stop eating snacks while watching TV or relaxing in another part of the house.

Category 2: 4 to 5 per day. Eat at least four to five small meals daily. Eating meals and planned snacks will stabilize your insulin levels and mobilize body fat to be burned during your exercise sessions.

Category 3: Eat less. By putting less food on your plate, you remove the temptation to overeat. Put one bite from your plate back into the serving dish before you sit down to eat.

Category 4: 1, 2, stop. Eat two morsels of food with proper chewing, then stop eating before the third bite and put your fork down. If you consume your meal in less than twenty minutes, your brain does not have a chance to get the message that you are being adequately nourished and you will feel hungry and frustrated. By eating slowly, you are sending a signal to the hypothalamus, the brain's thermostat, that food is in your system.

Category 5: Eight's too late. When you eat is also important. Never eat anything heavy later than eight o'clock because eating late does not allow your body time to utilize the calories. If you are hungry after eight, I suggest that you mix a tablespoon of whey protein powder into juice or water to increase your metabolic rate.

Category 6: No junk food between. Eating junk food calories between meals can add excess fat. Only eat appropriate snacks between meals.

Category 7: Never eat when upset. It is always best not to eat when under any type of stress, since you are not aware of what or of how much you are consuming when distracted by a stressor. Many people also eat the wrong types of foods—comfort foods such as desserts and pizza—when stressed.

Category 8: Proper rest. Obtaining seven to eight hours of sleep per night is a very important part of any successful nutritional or stress-reduction program. Night is your body's time for recuperation. Your kidneys also function best in a prone position. Make sure you are sound asleep before midnight to achieve the deep REM sleep state that truly relaxes your body and allows it to recuperate.

Category 9: Drink enough water. To give you the proper hydration level to keep your kidneys and your body's internal insulatory thermostat working properly so that you do not hoard fat, you should drink one-half to one ounce of water per pound of body weight per day. Water is one of your greatest allies in the business of weight loss.

Category 10: Intensity zone. You need to exercise in your gender-appropriate fat-burning zone on a regular basis.

Category 11: Brush your teeth. Brushing your teeth after each meal provides a sense of closure, changes the chemistry in your mouth, and reduces the urge to go back to the table and overeat.

Category 12: Visualize. Use visualization to see yourself achieving your fat-loss goals.

How to Score the Wellness Organizer

Review each of the twelve categories on a daily basis and give yourself 1 point for each one that you achieve. A perfect daily score is 12 and a perfect weekly score is 84. Don't be discouraged, however, if your first few weeks are less than perfect. Think of this as a tool to help you to see which areas you are strong in and which you need to work on and keep improving. Remember, you will only lose 2 pounds per week if you faithfully follow each step.

I have included a chart that you can photocopy to use over and over again.

	Sun.	Mon.	Tues.	Wed.	Thurs.	Fri.	Sat.	Sun.
1. Calories in the kitchen								
2. 4 to 5 per day								
3. Eat less								
4. 1, 2, stop								
5. Eight's too late								
6. No junk food between								
7. Never eat when upset								
8. Proper rest								
9. Drink enough water								
10. Intensity zone								
11. Brush your teeth								
12. Visualize								
Daily totals:								

The Four-Week Fat-Burning Program Guide

This four-week fat-loss program is meant to serve as a guide to help you get a strong start making the lifestyle changes described in this book. Following this program will help you create healthier routines and make them a part of your daily life. You should begin to see changes in your life such as more energy, a tighter and leaner body, increased strength and aerobic capacity, and greater peace of mind.

Don't be discouraged if you don't accomplish every task every day, or if you don't do every workout perfectly. The important thing is to improve, to make steady progress in substituting good habits for ones that do not serve you.

To begin, I'd like you to photocopy the following training log. Take a moment at the end of each day to check off each statement with a plus (+) or a minus (–). Your ultimate goal is a perfect score of 18 points.

TRAINING LOG

_____I ate three nutritious meals and two or three snacks today.

_____I chose only lean protein sources.

_____I chose complex carbohydrates over simple sugars.

_____I ate at least 25 grams of high-fiber foods such as oatmeal or a bran muffin.

_____I had at least five servings of fruits and vegetables today.

_____I avoided saturated fats and ate healthy monounsaturated fats.

_____I enjoyed whey protein powder as one of my snacks.

_____I drank one-half to one ounce of water per pound of body weight.

_____I did not have more than two cups of coffee or tea.

_____I avoided soft drinks containing sugar and caffeine.

_____I did not allow more than four hours between meals and snacks.

_____I understand that desserts are a special treat, so I skipped mine today.

_____I took my supplements, including my special fat-loss supplements.

_____I did not eat after eight o'clock at night.

_____I performed the appropriate exercise routine for the day.

_____I exercised at the proper level of intensity for my gender for each exercise.

_____I made time for myself today.

_____I utilized one of the gender-specific stress-handling techniques in chapter 7.

Number of points_____

Charts for Four-Week Fat-Burning Routines

I suggest making photocopies of these charts to help you keep track of your workout each day. For the circuit do either the gym routine or the home routine. Remember, during any single week you will be doing the circuit and steady-state cardio on days 1, 3, and 5 and the core exercises and interval training on days 2, 4, and 6. Make sure that you warm up for 5 or 10 minutes before doing the circuit and core exercises for 5 to 10 minutes, either by doing light calisthenics, stretches, or 5 minutes on the treadmill.

Gym Circuit	Repetitions	Gym Circuit	Repetitions
Chest Press	_____	Hip Adduction	_____
Leg Press	_____	Shoulder Press	_____
Seated Row	_____	Hip Abduction	_____
Leg Curl	_____	Abdominal Crunch	_____
Lateral Pull-down	_____	Back Extension	_____

Cardio Routine
Do the cardiovascular exercise of your choice, working to an ITT intensity level of 4–5.5 for men and 3.5–4.5 for women.

Home Circuit	Repetitions	Home Circuit	Repetitions
Push-ups	_____	Outer Thigh	_____
Wall Squat	_____	Lateral Raise	_____
Bent-over Row	_____	Inner Thigh	_____
Lunge	_____	Standard Crunch	_____
Shoulder Press	_____	Press-ups	_____

Cardio Routine

Do the cardiovascular exercise of your choice, working to an ITT intensity level of 4 to 5.5 for men and 3.5 to 4.5 for women.

Core Exercises	Repetitions	Core Exercises	Repetitions
Standard Crunch	_____	Superman or Superwoman	_____
Reverse Crunch	_____	Cross-Body Lift	_____
Oblique Crunch	_____	Back Raises	_____
Reverse Trunk Twist	_____	Side Twists	_____
Bridge	_____	Cat Stretch	_____

Interval Training

This is a suggested routine varying the intervals during each 20 seconds of active work. Begin by warming up for 10 minutes as described in chapter 13 at an IIT level of 3 to 4 for women and 4 to 5 for men.

		IIT Rate	
Work/Rest	Seconds	Women	Men
Work	20	6	7
Rest	40	3	4
Work	20	7	8
Rest	40	4	4
Work	20	8	9
Rest	40	4	5
Work	20	6	7
Rest	40	3	4
Work	20	7	8
Rest	40	3	4
Work	20	8	9
Rest	40	4	5
Work	20	6	7
Rest	40	3	4
Work	20	7	8
Rest	40	3	4
Work	20	8	9
Rest	40	4	5
Work	20	6	7
Rest	40	3	4

Remember to cool down for 10 minutes after you have completed your workout.

Day 1
Nutrition
Use the guidelines, meal plans, and recipes in chapters 8, 9, and 10 as a model. Also include the time that you ate each meal.

Breakfast _____

Snack _____

Lunch _____

Snack _____

Dinner _____

Snack _____

Daily fluid intake. Aim for one-half to one ounce per pound of body weight. Example: If you weigh 160 pounds, you should drink one and a half to three 1.5-liter bottles of water. _____

Coffee, tea, sodas. Always drink in moderation, since these contain caffeine and sugar. Most of your daily fluid intake should be water.

_____

Stress Management
Time spent doing some kind of activity to help minimize stress _____

Describe activity _____

Time spent journaling or doing something special for yourself _____

Daily Exercise
Don't forget to warm up and cool down for 10 minutes!
Time spent doing your circuit training (either the gym program or the at-home circuit program; the ideal is 10 minutes) _____

Number of circuits completed _____

Time spent doing cardio workout (the ideal is 50 minutes) _____

I stayed at my gender-appropriate level of intensity (always, mostly) _____

I kept my level of intensity steady-state throughout _____

How I felt at the end of my workout _____

End-of-Day Evaluation
Type of sleep (restful, restless)_____ How many hours _____

Stress levels (high, medium, low) _____

Level of energy (high, medium, low) _____

Significant accomplishments _____

Day 2
Nutrition
Use the guidelines, meal plans, and recipes in chapters 8, 9, and 10 as a model. Also include the time that you ate each meal.

Breakfast _____

Snack _____

Lunch _____

Snack _____

Dinner _____

Snack _____

Daily fluid intake. Aim for one-half to one ounce per pound of body weight. Example: If you weigh 160 pounds, you should drink one and a half to three 1.5-liter bottles of water. _____

Coffee, tea, sodas. Always drink in moderation, since these contain caffeine and sugar. Most of your daily fluid intake should be water.

_____

Stress Management
Time spent doing some kind of activity to help minimize stress _____

Describe activity _____

Time spent journaling or doing something special for yourself _____

Daily Exercise
Don't forget to warm up and cool down for 10 minutes!
Time spent doing core exercises (the ideal is 10 minutes) _____

Time spent doing interval training (the ideal time is 30 minutes) _____

I varied my level of intensity while staying within appropriate IIT Range for my gender _____

How I felt at the end of my workout _____

End-of-Day Evaluation
Type of sleep (restful, restless)____ How many hours _____

Stress levels (high, medium, low) _____

Level of energy (high, medium, low) _____

Significant accomplishments _____

Day 3
Nutrition
Use the guidelines, meal plans, and recipes in chapters 8, 9, and 10 as a model. Also include the time that you ate each meal.

Breakfast _____

Snack _____

Lunch _____

Snack _____

Dinner _____

Snack _____

Daily fluid intake. Aim for one-half to one ounce per pound of body weight. Example: If you weigh 160 pounds, you should drink one and a half to three 1.5-liter bottles of water. _____

Coffee, tea, sodas. Always drink in moderation, since these contain caffeine and sugar. Most of your daily fluid intake should be water.

Stress Management
Time spent doing some kind of activity to help minimize stress _____

Describe activity _____

Time spent journaling or doing something special for yourself _____

Daily Exercise
Don't forget to warm up and cool down for 10 minutes!
Time spent doing your circuit training (either the gym program or the at-home circuit program; the ideal is 10 minutes) _____

Number of circuits completed _____

Time spent doing cardio workout (the ideal is 50 minutes) _____

I stayed at my gender-appropriate level of intensity (always, mostly) _____

I kept my level of intensity steady-state throughout _____

How I felt at the end of my workout _____

End-of-Day Evaluation
Type of sleep (restful, restless)_____ How many hours _____

Stress levels (high, medium, low) _____

Level of energy (high, medium, low) _____

Significant accomplishments _____

Day 4
Nutrition
Use the guidelines, meal plans, and recipes in chapters 8, 9, and 10 as a model. Also include the time that you ate each meal.

Breakfast _____

Snack _____

Lunch _____

Snack _____

Dinner _____

Snack _____

Daily fluid intake. Aim for one-half to one ounce per pound of body weight. Example: If you weigh 160 pounds, you should drink one and a half to three 1.5-liter bottles of water. _____

Coffee, tea, sodas. Always drink in moderation, since these contain caffeine and sugar. Most of your daily fluid intake should be water.

Stress Management
Time spent doing some kind of activity to help minimize stress _____

Describe activity _____

Time spent journaling or doing something special for yourself _____

Daily Exercise
Don't forget to warm up and cool down for 10 minutes!
Time spent doing core exercises (the ideal is 10 minutes) _____

Time spent doing interval training (the ideal time is 30 minutes) _____

I varied my level of intensity while staying within appropriate IIT Range for my gender _____

How I felt at the end of my workout _____

End-of-Day Evaluation
Type of sleep (restful, restless)_____ How many hours _____

Stress levels (high, medium, low) _____

Level of energy (high, medium, low) _____

Significant accomplishments _____

Day 5
Nutrition

Use the guidelines, meal plans, and recipes in chapters 8, 9, and 10 as a model. Also include the time that you ate each meal.

Breakfast _____

Snack _____

Lunch _____

Snack _____

Dinner _____

Snack _____

Daily fluid intake. Aim for one-half to one ounce per pound of body weight. Example: If you weigh 160 pounds, you should drink one and a half to three 1.5-liter bottles of water. _____

Coffee, tea, sodas. Always drink in moderation, since these contain caffeine and sugar. Most of your daily fluid intake should be water.

_____

Stress Management

Time spent doing some kind of activity to help minimize stress _____

Describe activity _____

Time spent journaling or doing something special for yourself _____

Daily Exercise
Don't forget to warm up and cool down for 10 minutes!

Time spent doing your circuit training (either the gym program or the at-home circuit program; the ideal is 10 minutes) _____

Number of circuits completed _____

Time spent doing cardio workout (the ideal is 50 minutes) _____

I stayed at my gender-appropriate level of intensity (always, mostly) _____

I kept my level of intensity steady-state throughout _____

How I felt at the end of my workout _____

End-of-Day Evaluation

Type of sleep (restful, restless)_____ How many hours _____

Stress levels (high, medium, low) _____

Level of energy (high, medium, low) _____

Significant accomplishments _____

Day 6
Nutrition
Use the guidelines, meal plans, and recipes in chapters 8, 9, and 10 as a model. Also include the time that you ate each meal.

Breakfast _____

Snack _____

Lunch _____

Snack _____

Dinner _____

Snack _____

Daily fluid intake. Aim for one-half to one ounce per pound of body weight. Example: If you weigh 160 pounds, you should drink one and a half to three 1.5-liter bottles of water. _____

Coffee, tea, sodas. Always drink in moderation, since these contain caffeine and sugar. Most of your daily fluid intake should be water.

_____

Stress Management
Time spent doing some kind of activity to help minimize stress _____

Describe activity _____

Time spent journaling or doing something special for yourself _____

Daily Exercise
Don't forget to warm up and cool down for 10 minutes!
Time spent doing core exercises (the ideal is 10 minutes) _____

Time spent doing interval training (the ideal time is 30 minutes) _____

I varied my level of intensity while staying within appropriate IIT Range for my gender _____

How I felt at the end of my workout _____

End-of-Day Evaluation
Type of sleep (restful, restless)_____ How many hours _____

Stress levels (high, medium, low) _____

Level of energy (high, medium, low) _____

Significant accomplishments _____

Day 7
Nutrition
Use the guidelines, meal plans, and recipes in chapters 8, 9, and 10 as a model. Also include the time that you ate each meal.

Breakfast _____

Snack _____

Lunch _____

Snack _____

Dinner _____

Snack _____

Daily fluid intake. Aim for one-half to one ounce per pound of body weight. Example: If you weigh 160 pounds, you should drink one and a half to three 1.5-liter bottles of water. _____

Coffee, tea, sodas. Always drink in moderation, since these contain caffeine and sugar. Most of your daily fluid intake should be water.

Stress Management
Time spent doing some kind of activity to help minimize stress _____

Describe activity _____

Time spent journaling or doing something special for yourself _____

Daily Exercise
Don't forget to warm up and cool down for 10 minutes!
Time spent doing your circuit training (either the gym program or the at-home circuit program; the ideal is 10 minutes) _____

Number of circuits completed _____

Time spent doing cardio workout (the ideal is 50 minutes) _____

I stayed at my gender-appropriate level of intensity (always, mostly) ____

I kept my level of intensity steady-state throughout _____

How I felt at the end of my workout _____

End-of-Day Evaluation
Type of sleep (restful, restless)____ How many hours _____

Stress levels (high, medium, low) _____

Level of energy (high, medium, low) _____

Significant accomplishments _____

Day 8
Nutrition
Use the guidelines, meal plans, and recipes in chapters 8, 9, and 10 as a model. Also include the time that you ate each meal.

Breakfast _____

Snack _____

Lunch _____

Snack _____

Dinner _____

Snack _____

Daily fluid intake. Aim for one-half to one ounce per pound of body weight. Example: If you weigh 160 pounds, you should drink one and a half to three 1.5-liter bottles of water. _____

Coffee, tea, sodas. Always drink in moderation, since these contain caffeine and sugar. Most of your daily fluid intake should be water.

Stress Management
Time spent doing some kind of activity to help minimize stress _____

Describe activity _____

Time spent journaling or doing something special for yourself _____

Daily Exercise
Don't forget to warm up and cool down for 10 minutes!
Time spent doing core exercises (the ideal is 10 minutes) _____

Time spent doing interval training (the ideal time is 30 minutes) _____

I varied my level of intensity while staying within appropriate IIT Range for my gender _____

How I felt at the end of my workout _____

End-of-Day Evaluation
Type of sleep (restful, restless)_____ How many hours _____

Stress levels (high, medium, low) _____

Level of energy (high, medium, low) _____

Significant accomplishments _____

Day 9
Nutrition
Use the guidelines, meal plans, and recipes in chapters 8, 9, and 10 as a model. Also include the time that you ate each meal.

Breakfast _____

Snack _____

Lunch _____

Snack _____

Dinner _____

Snack _____

Daily fluid intake. Aim for one-half to one ounce per pound of body weight. Example: If you weigh 160 pounds, you should drink one and a half to three 1.5-liter bottles of water. _____

Coffee, tea, sodas. Always drink in moderation, since these contain caffeine and sugar. Most of your daily fluid intake should be water.

Stress Management
Time spent doing some kind of activity to help minimize stress _____

Describe activity _____

Time spent journaling or doing something special for yourself _____

Daily Exercise
Don't forget to warm up and cool down for 10 minutes!
Time spent doing your circuit training (either the gym program or the at-home circuit program; the ideal is 10 minutes) _____

Number of circuits completed _____

Time spent doing cardio workout (the ideal is 50 minutes) _____

I stayed at my gender-appropriate level of intensity (always, mostly) _____

I kept my level of intensity steady-state throughout _____

How I felt at the end of my workout _____

End-of-Day Evaluation
Type of sleep (restful, restless)_____ How many hours _____

Stress levels (high, medium, low) _____

Level of energy (high, medium, low) _____

Significant accomplishments _____

Day 10
Nutrition
Use the guidelines, meal plans, and recipes in chapters 8, 9, and 10 as a model. Also include the time that you ate each meal.

Breakfast _____

Snack _____

Lunch _____

Snack _____

Dinner _____

Snack _____

Daily fluid intake. Aim for one-half to one ounce per pound of body weight. Example: If you weigh 160 pounds, you should drink one and a half to three 1.5-liter bottles of water. _____

Coffee, tea, sodas. Always drink in moderation, since these contain caffeine and sugar. Most of your daily fluid intake should be water.

_____

Stress Management
Time spent doing some kind of activity to help minimize stress _____

Describe activity _____

Time spent journaling or doing something special for yourself _____

Daily Exercise
Don't forget to warm up and cool down for 10 minutes!
Time spent doing core exercises (the ideal is 10 minutes) _____

Time spent doing interval training (the ideal time is 30 minutes) _____

I varied my level of intensity while staying within appropriate IIT Range for my gender _____

How I felt at the end of my workout _____

End-of-Day Evaluation
Type of sleep (restful, restless)_____ How many hours _____

Stress levels (high, medium, low) _____

Level of energy (high, medium, low) _____

Significant accomplishments _____

Day 11
Nutrition
Use the guidelines, meal plans, and recipes in chapters 8, 9, and 10 as a model. Also include the time that you ate each meal.

Breakfast _____

Snack _____

Lunch _____

Snack _____

Dinner _____

Snack _____

Daily fluid intake. Aim for one-half to one ounce per pound of body weight. Example: If you weigh 160 pounds, you should drink one and a half to three 1.5-liter bottles of water. _____

Coffee, tea, sodas. Always drink in moderation, since these contain caffeine and sugar. Most of your daily fluid intake should be water.

_____

Stress Management
Time spent doing some kind of activity to help minimize stress _____
Describe activity _____
Time spent journaling or doing something special for yourself _____

Daily Exercise
Don't forget to warm up and cool down for 10 minutes!
Time spent doing circuit training (either the gym program or the at-home circuit program; the ideal is 10 minutes) _____

Number of circuits completed _____

Time spent doing cardio workout (the ideal is 50 minutes) _____

I stayed at my gender-appropriate level of intensity (always, mostly) ____

I kept my level of intensity steady-state throughout _____

How I felt at the end of my workout _____

End-of-Day Evaluation
Type of sleep (restful, restless)____ How many hours _____

Stress levels (high, medium, low) _____

Level of energy (high, medium, low) _____

Significant accomplishments _____

Day 12
Nutrition
Use the guidelines, meal plans, and recipes in chapters 8, 9, and 10 as a model. Also include the time that you ate each meal.

Breakfast _____

Snack _____

Lunch _____

Snack _____

Dinner _____

Snack _____

Daily fluid intake. Aim for one-half to one ounce per pound of body weight. Example: If you weigh 160 pounds, you should drink one and a half to three 1.5-liter bottles of water. _____

Coffee, tea, sodas. Always drink in moderation, since these contain caffeine and sugar. Most of your daily fluid intake should be water.

_____

Stress Management
Time spent doing some kind of activity to help minimize stress _____

Describe activity _____

Time spent journaling or doing something special for yourself _____

Daily Exercise
Don't forget to warm up and cool down for 10 minutes!
Time spent doing core exercises (the ideal is 10 minutes) _____

Time spent doing interval training (the ideal time is 30 minutes) _____

I varied my level of intensity while staying within appropriate IIT Range for my gender _____

How I felt at the end of my workout _____

End-of-Day Evaluation
Type of sleep (restful, restless)_____ How many hours _____

Stress levels (high, medium, low) _____

Level of energy (high, medium, low) _____

Significant accomplishments _____

Day 13
Nutrition
Use the guidelines, meal plans, and recipes in chapters 8, 9, and 10 as a model. Also include the time that you ate each meal.

Breakfast _____

Snack _____

Lunch _____

Snack _____

Dinner _____

Snack _____

Daily fluid intake. Aim for one-half to one ounce per pound of body weight. Example: If you weigh 160 pounds, you should drink one and a half to three 1.5-liter bottles of water. _____

Coffee, tea, sodas. Always drink in moderation, since these contain caffeine and sugar. Most of your daily fluid intake should be water.

_____

Stress Management
Time spent doing some kind of activity to help minimize stress _____

Describe activity _____

Time spent journaling or doing something special for yourself _____

Daily Exercise
Don't forget to warm up and cool down for 10 minutes!
Time spent doing your circuit training (either the gym program or the at-home circuit program; the ideal is 10 minutes) _____

Number of circuits completed _____

Time spent doing cardio workout (the ideal is 50 minutes) _____

I stayed at my gender-appropriate level of intensity (always, mostly) _____

I kept my level of intensity steady-state throughout _____

How I felt at the end of my workout _____

End-of-Day Evaluation
Type of sleep (restful, restless)_____ How many hours _____

Stress levels (high, medium, low) _____

Level of energy (high, medium, low) _____

Significant accomplishments _____

Day 14
Nutrition
Use the guidelines, meal plans, and recipes in chapters 8, 9, and 10 as a model. Also include the time that you ate each meal.

Breakfast _____

Snack _____

Lunch _____

Snack _____

Dinner _____

Snack _____

Daily fluid intake. Aim for one-half to one ounce per pound of body weight. Example: If you weigh 160 pounds, you should drink one and a half to three 1.5-liter bottles of water. _____

Coffee, tea, sodas. Always drink in moderation, since these contain caffeine and sugar. Most of your daily fluid intake should be water.

_____

Stress Management
Time spent doing some kind of activity to help minimize stress _____

Describe activity _____

Time spent journaling or doing something special for yourself _____

Daily Exercise
Don't forget to warm up and cool down for 10 minutes!
Time spent doing core exercises (the ideal is 10 minutes) _____

Time spent doing interval training (the ideal time is 30 minutes) _____

I varied my level of intensity while staying within appropriate IIT Range for my gender _____

How I felt at the end of my workout _____

End-of-Day Evaluation
Type of sleep (restful, restless)_____ How many hours _____

Stress levels (high, medium, low) _____

Level of energy (high, medium, low) _____

Significant accomplishments _____

Day 15
Nutrition

Use the guidelines, meal plans, and recipes in chapters 8, 9, and 10 as a model. Also include the time that you ate each meal.

Breakfast _____

Snack _____

Lunch _____

Snack _____

Dinner _____

Snack _____

Daily fluid intake. Aim for one-half to one ounce per pound of body weight. Example: If you weigh 160 pounds, you should drink one and a half to three 1.5-liter bottles of water. _____

Coffee, tea, sodas. Always drink in moderation, since these contain caffeine and sugar. Most of your daily fluid intake should be water.

_____

Stress Management

Time spent doing some kind of activity to help minimize stress _____

Describe activity _____

Time spent journaling or doing something special for yourself _____

Daily Exercise

Don't forget to warm up and cool down for 10 minutes!

Time spent doing your circuit training (either the gym program or the at-home circuit program; the ideal is 10 minutes) _____

Number of circuits completed _____

Time spent doing cardio workout (the ideal is 50 minutes) _____

I stayed at my gender-appropriate level of intensity (always, mostly) _____

I kept my level of intensity steady-state throughout _____

How I felt at the end of my workout _____

End-of-Day Evaluation

Type of sleep (restful, restless)_____ How many hours _____

Stress levels (high, medium, low) _____

Level of energy (high, medium, low) _____

Significant accomplishments _____

Day 16
Nutrition

Use the guidelines, meal plans, and recipes in chapters 8, 9, and 10 as a model. Also include the time that you ate each meal.

Breakfast _____

Snack _____

Lunch _____

Snack _____

Dinner _____

Snack _____

Daily fluid intake. Aim for one-half to one ounce per pound of body weight. Example: If you weigh 160 pounds, you should drink one and a half to three 1.5-liter bottles of water. _____

Coffee, tea, sodas. Always drink in moderation, since these contain caffeine and sugar. Most of your daily fluid intake should be water.

_____

Stress Management

Time spent doing some kind of activity to help minimize stress _____

Describe activity _____

Time spent journaling or doing something special for yourself _____

Daily Exercise
Don't forget to warm up and cool down for 10 minutes!

Time spent doing core exercises (the ideal is 10 minutes) _____

Time spent doing interval training (the ideal time is 30 minutes) _____

I varied my level of intensity while staying within appropriate IIT Range for my gender _____

How I felt at the end of my workout _____

End-of-Day Evaluation

Type of sleep (restful, restless)_____ How many hours _____

Stress levels (high, medium, low) _____

Level of energy (high, medium, low) _____

Significant accomplishments _____

Day 17
Nutrition
Use the guidelines, meal plans, and recipes in chapters 8, 9, and 10 as a model. Also include the time that you ate each meal.

Breakfast _____

Snack _____

Lunch _____

Snack _____

Dinner _____

Snack _____

Daily fluid intake. Aim for one-half to one ounce per pound of body weight. Example: If you weigh 160 pounds, you should drink one and a half to three 1.5-liter bottles of water. _____

Coffee, tea, sodas. Always drink in moderation, since these contain caffeine and sugar. Most of your daily fluid intake should be water.

Stress Management
Time spent doing some kind of activity to help minimize stress _____

Describe activity _____

Time spent journaling or doing something special for yourself _____

Daily Exercise
Don't forget to warm up and cool down for 10 minutes!
Time spent doing your circuit training (either the gym program or the at-home circuit program; the ideal is 10 minutes) _____

Number of circuits completed _____

Time spent doing cardio workout (the ideal is 50 minutes) _____

I stayed at my gender-appropriate level of intensity (always, mostly) ____

I kept my level of intensity steady-state throughout _____

How I felt at the end of my workout _____

End-of-Day Evaluation
Type of sleep (restful, restless)____ How many hours _____

Stress levels (high, medium, low) _____

Level of energy (high, medium, low) _____

Significant accomplishments _____

Day 18
Nutrition
Use the guidelines, meal plans, and recipes in chapters 8, 9, and 10 as a model. Also include the time that you ate each meal.

Breakfast _____

Snack _____

Lunch _____

Snack _____

Dinner _____

Snack _____

Daily fluid intake. Aim for one-half to one ounce per pound of body weight. Example: If you weigh 160 pounds, you should drink one and a half to three 1.5-liter bottles of water. _____

Coffee, tea, sodas. Always drink in moderation, since these contain caffeine and sugar. Most of your daily fluid intake should be water.

_____

Stress Management
Time spent doing some kind of activity to help minimize stress _____

Describe activity _____

Time spent journaling or doing something special for yourself _____

Daily Exercise
Don't forget to warm up and cool down for 10 minutes!
Time spent doing core exercises (the ideal is 10 minutes) _____

Time spent doing interval training (the ideal time is 30 minutes) _____

I varied my level of intensity while staying within appropriate IIT Range for my gender _____

How I felt at the end of my workout _____

End-of-Day Evaluation
Type of sleep (restful, restless) _____ How many hours _____

Stress levels (high, medium, low) _____

Level of energy (high, medium, low) _____

Significant accomplishments _____

Day 19
Nutrition
Use the guidelines, meal plans, and recipes in chapters 8, 9, and 10 as a model. Also include the time that you ate each meal.

Breakfast _____

Snack _____

Lunch _____

Snack _____

Dinner _____

Snack _____

Daily fluid intake. Aim for one-half to one ounce per pound of body weight. Example: If you weigh 160 pounds, you should drink one and a half to three 1.5-liter bottles of water. _____

Coffee, tea, sodas. Always drink in moderation, since these contain caffeine and sugar. Most of your daily fluid intake should be water.

_____

Stress Management
Time spent doing some kind of activity to help minimize stress _____

Describe activity _____

Time spent journaling or doing something special for yourself _____

Daily Exercise
Don't forget to warm up and cool down for 10 minutes!
Time spent doing your circuit training (either the gym program or the at-home circuit program; the ideal is 10 minutes) _____

Number of circuits completed _____

Time spent doing cardio workout (the ideal is 50 minutes) _____

I stayed at my gender-appropriate level of intensity (always, mostly) _____

I kept my level of intensity steady-state throughout _____

How I felt at the end of my workout _____

End-of-Day Evaluation
Type of sleep (restful, restless)_____ How many hours _____

Stress levels (high, medium, low) _____

Level of energy (high, medium, low) _____

Significant accomplishments _____

Day 20
Nutrition
Use the guidelines, meal plans, and recipes in chapters 8, 9, and 10 as a model. Also include the time that you ate each meal.

Breakfast _____

Snack _____

Lunch _____

Snack _____

Dinner _____

Snack _____

Daily fluid intake. Aim for one-half to one ounce per pound of body weight. Example: If you weigh 160 pounds, you should drink one and a half to three 1.5-liter bottles of water. _____

Coffee, tea, sodas. Always drink in moderation, since these contain caffeine and sugar. Most of your daily fluid intake should be water.

Stress Management
Time spent doing some kind of activity to help minimize stress _____

Describe activity _____

Time spent journaling or doing something special for yourself _____

Daily Exercise
Don't forget to warm up and cool down for 10 minutes!
Time spent doing core exercises (the ideal is 10 minutes) _____

Time spent doing interval training (the ideal time is 30 minutes) _____

I varied my level of intensity while staying within appropriate IIT Range for my gender _____

How I felt at the end of my workout _____

End-of-Day Evaluation
Type of sleep (restful, restless)_____ How many hours _____

Stress levels (high, medium, low) _____

Level of energy (high, medium, low) _____

Significant accomplishments _____

Day 21
Nutrition
Use the guidelines, meal plans, and recipes in chapters 8, 9, and 10 as a model. Also include the time that you ate each meal.

Breakfast _____

Snack _____

Lunch _____

Snack _____

Dinner _____

Snack _____

Daily fluid intake. Aim for one-half to one ounce per pound of body weight. Example: If you weigh 160 pounds, you should drink one and a half to three 1.5-liter bottles of water. _____

Coffee, tea, sodas. Always drink in moderation, since these contain caffeine and sugar. Most of your daily fluid intake should be water.

Stress Management
Time spent doing some kind of activity to help minimize stress _____

Describe activity _____

Time spent journaling or doing something special for yourself _____

Daily Exercise
Don't forget to warm up and cool down for 10 minutes!
Time spent doing your circuit training (either the gym program or the at-home circuit program; the ideal is 10 minutes) _____

Number of circuits completed _____

Time spent doing cardio workout (the ideal is 50 minutes) _____

I stayed at my gender-appropriate level of intensity (always, mostly) _____

I kept my level of intensity steady-state throughout _____

How I felt at the end of my workout _____

End-of-Day Evaluation
Type of sleep (restful, restless)_____ How many hours _____

Stress levels (high, medium, low) _____

Level of energy (high, medium, low) _____

Significant accomplishments _____

Day 22
Nutrition

Use the guidelines, meal plans, and recipes in chapters 8, 9, and 10 as a model. Also include the time that you ate each meal.

Breakfast _____

Snack _____

Lunch _____

Snack _____

Dinner _____

Snack _____

Daily fluid intake. Aim for one-half to one ounce per pound of body weight. Example: If you weigh 160 pounds, you should drink one and a half to three 1.5-liter bottles of water. _____

Coffee, tea, sodas. Always drink in moderation, since these contain caffeine and sugar. Most of your daily fluid intake should be water.

Stress Management

Time spent doing some kind of activity to help minimize stress _____

Describe activity _____

Time spent journaling or doing something special for yourself _____

Daily Exercise

Don't forget to warm up and cool down for 10 minutes!

Time spent doing core exercises (the ideal is 10 minutes) _____

Time spent doing interval training (the ideal time is 30 minutes) _____

I varied my level of intensity while staying within appropriate IIT Range for my gender _____

How I felt at the end of my workout _____

End-of-Day Evaluation

Type of sleep (restful, restless)____ How many hours _____

Stress levels (high, medium, low) _____

Level of energy (high, medium, low) _____

Significant accomplishments _____

Day 23
Nutrition

Use the guidelines, meal plans, and recipes in chapters 8, 9, and 10 as a model. Also include the time that you ate each meal.

Breakfast _____

Snack _____

Lunch _____

Snack _____

Dinner _____

Snack _____

Daily fluid intake. Aim for one-half to one ounce per pound of body weight. Example: If you weigh 160 pounds, you should drink one and a half to three 1.5-liter bottles of water. _____

Coffee, tea, sodas. Always drink in moderation, since these contain caffeine and sugar. Most of your daily fluid intake should be water.

_____

Stress Management

Time spent doing some kind of activity to help minimize stress _____

Describe activity _____

Time spent journaling or doing something special for yourself _____

Daily Exercise

Don't forget to warm up and cool down for 10 minutes!

Time spent doing your circuit training (either the gym program or the at-home circuit program; the ideal is 10 minutes) _____

Number of circuits completed _____

Time spent doing cardio workout (the ideal is 50 minutes) _____

I stayed at my gender-appropriate level of intensity (always, mostly) _____

I kept my level of intensity steady-state throughout _____

How I felt at the end of my workout _____

End-of-Day Evaluation

Type of sleep (restful, restless)_____ How many hours _____

Stress levels (high, medium, low) _____

Level of energy (high, medium, low) _____

Significant accomplishments _____

Day 24
Nutrition
Use the guidelines, meal plans, and recipes in chapters 8, 9, and 10 as a model. Also include the time that you ate each meal.

Breakfast _____

Snack _____

Lunch _____

Snack _____

Dinner _____

Snack _____

Daily fluid intake. Aim for one-half to one ounce per pound of body weight. Example: If you weigh 160 pounds, you should drink one and a half to three 1.5-liter bottles of water. _____

Coffee, tea, sodas. Always drink in moderation, since these contain caffeine and sugar. Most of your daily fluid intake should be water.

Stress Management
Time spent doing some kind of activity to help minimize stress _____

Describe activity _____

Time spent journaling or doing something special for yourself _____

Daily Exercise
Don't forget to warm up and cool down for 10 minutes!
Time spent doing core exercises (the ideal is 10 minutes) _____

Time spent doing interval training (the ideal time is 30 minutes) _____

I varied my level of intensity while staying within appropriate IIT Range for my gender _____

How I felt at the end of my workout _____

End-of-Day Evaluation
Type of sleep (restful, restless)_____ How many hours _____

Stress levels (high, medium, low) _____

Level of energy (high, medium, low) _____

Significant accomplishments _____

Day 25
Nutrition
Use the guidelines, meal plans, and recipes in chapters 8, 9, and 10 as a model. Also include the time that you ate each meal.

Breakfast _____

Snack _____

Lunch _____

Snack _____

Dinner _____

Snack _____

Daily fluid intake. Aim for one-half to one ounce per pound of body weight. Example: If you weigh 160 pounds, you should drink one and a half to three 1.5-liter bottles of water. _____

Coffee, tea, sodas. Always drink in moderation, since these contain caffeine and sugar. Most of your daily fluid intake should be water.

Stress Management
Time spent doing some kind of activity to help minimize stress _____

Describe activity _____

Time spent journaling or doing something special for yourself _____

Daily Exercise
Don't forget to warm up and cool down for 10 minutes!
Time spent doing your circuit training (either the gym program or the at-home circuit program; the ideal is 10 minutes) _____

Number of circuits completed _____

Time spent doing cardio workout (the ideal is 50 minutes) _____

I stayed at my gender-appropriate level of intensity (always, mostly) _____

I kept my level of intensity steady-state throughout _____

How I felt at the end of my workout _____

End-of-Day Evaluation
Type of sleep (restful, restless)_____ How many hours _____

Stress levels (high, medium, low) _____

Level of energy (high, medium, low) _____

Significant accomplishments _____

Day 26
Nutrition
Use the guidelines, meal plans, and recipes in chapters 8, 9, and 10 as a model. Also include the time that you ate each meal.

Breakfast _____

Snack _____

Lunch _____

Snack _____

Dinner _____

Snack _____

Daily fluid intake. Aim for one-half to one ounce per pound of body weight. Example: If you weigh 160 pounds, you should drink one and a half to three 1.5-liter bottles of water. _____

Coffee, tea, sodas. Always drink in moderation, since these contain caffeine and sugar. Most of your daily fluid intake should be water.

Stress Management
Time spent doing some kind of activity to help minimize stress _____

Describe activity _____

Time spent journaling or doing something special for yourself _____

Daily Exercise
Don't forget to warm up and cool down for 10 minutes!
Time spent doing core exercises (the ideal is 10 minutes) _____

Time spent doing interval training (the ideal time is 30 minutes) _____

I varied my level of intensity while staying within appropriate IIT Range for my gender _____

How I felt at the end of my workout _____

End-of-Day Evaluation
Type of sleep (restful, restless)____ How many hours _____

Stress levels (high, medium, low) _____

Level of energy (high, medium, low) _____

Significant accomplishments _____

Day 27
Nutrition
Use the guidelines, meal plans, and recipes in chapters 8, 9, and 10 as a model. Also include the time that you ate each meal.

Breakfast _____

Snack _____

Lunch _____

Snack _____

Dinner _____

Snack _____

Daily fluid intake. Aim for one-half to one ounce per pound of body weight. Example: If you weigh 160 pounds, you should drink one and a half to three 1.5-liter bottles of water. _____

Coffee, tea, sodas. Always drink in moderation, since these contain caffeine and sugar. Most of your daily fluid intake should be water.

Stress Management
Time spent doing some kind of activity to help minimize stress _____

Describe activity _____

Time spent journaling or doing something special for yourself _____

Daily Exercise
Don't forget to warm up and cool down for 10 minutes!
Time spent doing your circuit training (either the gym program or the at-home circuit program; the ideal is 10 minutes) _____

Number of circuits completed _____

Time spent doing cardio workout (the ideal is 50 minutes) _____

I stayed at my gender-appropriate level of intensity (always, mostly) _____

I kept my level of intensity steady-state throughout _____

How I felt at the end of my workout _____

End-of-Day Evaluation
Type of sleep (restful, restless)_____ How many hours _____

Stress levels (high, medium, low) _____

Level of energy (high, medium, low) _____

Significant accomplishments _____

Day 28
Nutrition

Use the guidelines, meal plans, and recipes in chapters 8, 9, and 10 as a model. Also include the time that you ate each meal.

Breakfast _____

Snack _____

Lunch _____

Snack _____

Dinner _____

Snack _____

Daily fluid intake. Aim for one-half to one ounce per pound of body weight. Example: If you weigh 160 pounds, you should drink one and a half to three 1.5-liter bottles of water. _____

Coffee, tea, sodas. Always drink in moderation, since these contain caffeine and sugar. Most of your daily fluid intake should be water.

Stress Management

Time spent doing some kind of activity to help minimize stress _____

Describe activity _____

Time spent journaling or doing something special for yourself _____

Daily Exercise
Don't forget to warm up and cool down for 10 minutes!

Time spent doing core exercises (the ideal is 10 minutes) _____

Time spent doing interval training (the ideal time is 30 minutes) _____

I varied my level of intensity while staying within appropriate IIT Range for my gender _____

How I felt at the end of my workout _____

End-of-Day Evaluation

Type of sleep (restful, restless)_____ How many hours _____

Stress levels (high, medium, low) _____

Level of energy (high, medium, low) _____

Significant accomplishments _____

Resources to Help You

Medical Organizations

American Academy of Family
    Physicians
11400 Tomahawk Creek Parkway
Leawood, KS 66211-2672
www.familydoctor.org

American Heart Association (AHA)
National Center
7272 Greenville Avenue
Dallas, TX 75231
800-242-8721
www.americanheart.org

Centers for Disease Control and
    Prevention
National Center for Chronic Disease
    Prevention and Health Promotion
Division of Nutrition and Physical
    Activity
4770 Buford Highway NE
Atlanta, GA 30341
770-488-5820
www.cdc.gov/nccdphp/dnpa

National Cholesterol Education
    Program
NHLBI Health Information Center
P.O. Box 30105
Bethesda, MD 20824-0105
301-592-8573
www.nhlbi.nih.gov/about/ncep

National Mental Health Association
2001 North Beauregard Street,
    12th Floor
Alexandria, VA 22311
800-969-NMHA
www.nmha.org

Nutrition Organizations

American Dietetic Association (ADA)
216 West Jackson Boulevard
Chicago, IL 60606-6995
800-877-1600; 312-899-0040
800-366-1655 (consumer hotline)
e-mail: hotline@eatright.org;
    infocenter@eatright.org

American Society for Clinical Nutrition
    (ASCN)
9650 Rockville Pike
Bethesda, MD 20814
301-530-7110
e-mail: secretar@acsn.faseb.org

Glycemic Research Institute
601 Pennsylvania Avenue NW, Suite 900
Washington, DC 20004
202-434-8270
www.glycemic.com
www.anndeweesallen.com

U.S. Food and Drug Administration
5600 Fishers Lane
Rockville, MD 20857-0001
888-463-6332
www.fda.gov

Fitness Organizations

American College of Sports Medicine
    (ACSM)
401 West Michigan Street
Indianapolis, IN 46206-3233
317-637-9200
www.acsm.org

American Council on Exercise (ACE)
5820 Oberlin Drive, Suite 102
San Diego, CA 92121-3787
619-535-8227
www.acefitness.org

Cooper Institute for Aerobic Research
  (CIAR)
12330 Preston Road
Dallas, TX 75230
214-701-8001
www.cooperinst.org

National Women's Health Information
  Center
8550 Arlington Boulevard, Suite 300
Fairfax, VA 22031
800-994-9662

800-220-5446 (TDD)
www.4woman.gov/fag/heartdise.htm

President's Council on Physical Fitness
  and Sports
Hubert H. Humphrey Building, Room
  738-H
200 Independence Avenue SW
Washington, DC 20201-0004
202-690-9000
www.fitness.gov

Shape Up America!
6707 Democracy Boulevard, Suite 306
Bethesda, MD 20817
301-493-5368
www.shapeup.org

Books

Barnes, Broda. *Hyperthyroidism, the Unsuspected Illness.* New York: HarperCollins, 1976.

Brand-Miller, J., Thomas M. S. Wolever, and Kaye Foster-Powell. *The Glucose Revolution: The Authoritative Guide to the Glycemic Index.* New York: Marlowe and Co., 1999.

Castelli, William P., and Glen C. Griffin. *Good Fat, Bad Fat: How to Lower Your Cholesterol and Reduce the Odds of a Heart Attack.* Tucson, Ariz.: Fisher Books, 1997.

Charnetski, Carl J., and Francis X. Brennan. *Feeling Good Is Good for You: How Pleasure Can Boost Your Immune System and Lengthen Your Life.* New York: Rodale, 2001.

Cowden, W. Lee, Ferre Akbarpour, Russ Dicarlo, and Burton Goldberg. *Longevity: Reverse the Aging Process and Stay Young with Clinically Proven Alternative Therapies.* Alternative Medicine.com, Inc., 2001.

De Orio, Keith, with Robert Dursi. *The New Millennium Diet Revolution.* New York: Prominence Publishers, 2000.

Domar, Alice. *Self-Nurture: Learning to Care for Yourself as Effectively as You Care for Everyone Else.* New York: Penguin, 2001.

Goglia, Philip L. *Turn Up the Heat: Unlock the Fat-Burning Power of Your Metabolism.* New York: Viking, 2002.

Milnor, J. Pervis III, et al. *It Can Break Your Heart: What You and Your Doctor Should Know about Your Weight Problem.* New York: Eagle Wing Books, 2000.

Murray, Michael T. *Dr. Murray's Total Body Tune-up*. New York: Bantam, 2000.

Peeke, Pamela. *Fight Fat after Forty*. New York: Viking Press, 2000.

Shilstone, Mackie. *Lose Your Love Handles: A 3-Step Program to Stream-line Your Waist in 30 Days*. New York: Perigee, 2001.

———. *Maximum Energy for Life: A 21-Day Strategic Plan to Feel Great, Reverse the Aging Process, and Optimize Your Health*. Hoboken, N.J.: John Wiley & Sons, 2003.

Willis, Clint, ed. *Why Meditate? The Essential Book about How Medita-tion Can Enrich Your Life*. New York: Marlowe and Company, 2001.

Wise, Anna. *The High Performance Mind: Mastering Brainwaves for Insight, Healing, and Creativity*. New York: Tarcher Putnam, 1995.

Health Journals

Canadian Journal of Applied
    Physiology
Human Kinetics Publishers, Inc.
P.O. Box 5076
Champaign, IL 61825-5076
800-747-4457
www.humankinetics.com

Exercise and Sports Sciences
    Reviews
American College of Sports
    Medicine
P.O. Box 1550
Hagerstown, MD 21740
800-638-3030
www.medscape.com

Functional Medicine Update:
The Voice of Functional and
    Nutritional Medicine
P.O. Box 1697
Gig Harbor, WA 98335
800-228-0622
www.functionalmedicine.org

International Journal of Sport Nutrition
    and Exercise Metabolism
Human Kinetics Publishers, Inc.
P.O. Box 5076
Champaign, IL 61825-5076
800-747-4457
www.humankinetics.com

Journal of Nutritional Biochemistry
360 Park Avenue South
New York, NY 10010-1710
877-839-7126
www.elsevier.com

Journal of Sport Rehabilitation
Human Kinetics Publishers, Inc.
P.O. Box 5076
Champaign, IL 61825-5076
800-747-4457
www.humankinetics.com

Let's Live Magazine
P.O. Box 74908
Los Angeles, CA 90004
800-676-4333
www.Letsliveonline.com

Medicine and Science in Sports and
    Exercise:
Official Journal of the American College
    of Sports Medicine
American College of Sports Medicine
401 West Michigan Street
Indianapolis, IN 46202-3233
317-637-9200
www.acsm-msse.org

Strength and Conditioning Journal
1885 Bob Johnson Drive
Colorado Springs, CO 80906
719-632-6722
www.nsca-lift.org

Additional Online Resources

American Dietetic Association
www.eatright.org

Center for Anxiety and Stress Treatment
www.stressrelease.com

Health Net
www.healthnet.com

Institute for Stress Management
www.hyperstress.com

My Personal Web Page
www.mackieshilstone.com

Thyroid Information
doctors@MaryClinic.com

Ochsner Clinic Foundation
www.ochsner.org

Omega Institute for Holistic Studies
www.omega-inst.org

Heart Health Evaluation
www.myheartrisk.com

Purchase Soy Products Online
www.revivalsoy.com

Yoga Journal
www.yogajournal.com

*on*health
www.onhealth.com

Books and Workshops for Stress
Management
www.Ihaveavoice.com

General Medical Information and
Services
www.WebMD.com

Dietary Approaches to Stopping
Hypertension (DASH)
www.nhlbi.nih.gov/health/public/
heart/hbp/dash/

Nurses Health Study
www.womens-health.org

American Diabetes Association
www.diabetes.org/home.jsp

Women's Health Initiative
www.nhlbi.nih.gov/whi.org and
www.delay-ad.org

U.S. Physicians Health Study
phs.bwh.harvard.edu/pubs.htm

Index